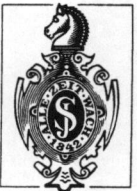

E. Gladtke · H. M. von Hattingberg

Pharmacokinetics

An Introduction

With Contributions by W. Kübler, W.-H. Wagner
and a Foreword by E. R. Garrett

Translated by P. J. Wilkinson

With 72 Figures

Springer-Verlag
Berlin · Heidelberg · New York 1979

Prof. Dr. E. GLADTKE, Direktor der Universitäts-Kinderklinik, Josef-Stelzmann-Straße 9, D-5000 Köln 41

Prof. Dr. H. M. von HATTINGBERG, Kinderklinik der Justus-Liebig-Universität, Klinikstraße 28, D-6300 Gießen

Prof. Dr. W. KÜBLER, Institut für Ernährungswissenschaft I der Justus-Liebig-Universität, Goethestraße 55, D-6300 Gießen

Prof. Dr. W.-H. WAGNER, Farbwerke Hoechst AG, Arbeitsgruppe Chemotherapie, Postfach 800320, D-6230 Frankfurt 80

Translator
Dr. P. Wilkinson, M. A., M. B., M. R. C. Path., Consultant Senior Lecturer in Clinical, Bacteriology. Dept. of Microbiology, Bristol Health District (Teaching), Bristol Royal Infirmary, Bristol BS2 8HW, Great Britain

ISBN-13:978-3-540-09183-7   e-ISBN-13:978-3-642-67188-3
DOI: 10.1007/978-3-642-67188-3

Library of Congress Cataloging in Publication Data. Gladtke, Erich. Pharmacokinetics: an introduction. Translation of the 2d rev. ed. of Pharmakokinetik. Bibliography: p. .Includes index. 1. Pharmacokinetics. I. Hattingberg, H. M. von, joint author. II. Title. [DNLM: 1. Pharmacology. QV38.3 G542p]. RM301.5.G5513. 615'.7. 78-26961.

This work is subject to copyright. All rights are reserved, whether the whole or part of the material is concerned specifically those of translation, reprinting. re-use of illustrations, broadcasting, reproduction by photocopying machine or similar means, and storage in data banks. Under § 54 of the German Law where copies are made for other than private use, a fee is payable to the publisher, the amount of the fee to be determined by agreement with the publisher.

© by Springer-Verlag Berlin Heidelberg 1979

The use of registered names, trademarks, etc. in this publication does not imply, even in the absence of a specific statement, that such names are exempt from the relevant protective laws and regulations and therefore free for general use.

Foreword

This is a little book with no great pretensions. The authors do not claim it to be world-startling nor Nobel- or Pulitzer-prize-winning. It is a valuable primer for pharmacokinetics for those desiring a proper initiation into previously assumed mysteries. It is fully intended as an introduction to the basic concept of pharmacokinetics and will be welcomed by all who wish to apply its principles to their own disciplines, whether in life sciences or medicine, without being confused by excess mathematics.

It is edited by two well-known German scientists who are primarily practicing pediatricians and who use pharmacokinetics in their daily work, in a field of medicine where the proper adjustment of doses for infants and children is a delicate and life-preserving art. They were trained as pediatricians *and* as pharmacokinetists by the world-renowned Professor F. HARTMUT DOST, who uniquely synthesized these two disciplines and who, as a pioneer in this field, published the first book on pharmacokinetics in 1953. In their own right, the editors have conducted excellent and unique research on the effect and fate of drugs and have followed up the unexpected changes in drug action accompanying the rapid developments encountered in the initial hours, days, and weeks after birth.

You will find some interesting Germanisms in this book à la Professor DOST. I personally feel that these will give some spice to their renditions. For example, the use of the term "invasion" to represent the transfer of a substance from a compartment of entry to a compartment from which blood is drawn for analysis is a purely German term that does not exist in American or English publications on pharmacokinetics. Nevertheless, such terms are well defined in the text and may become common usage in the English-speaking world.

Last but not least, I must state that the editors of this book are my personal friends. I do not believe that this fact has obscured my evaluation of their manuscript. In fact, it enables me to tell you more about the personalities behind the words. They are warm human beings who have faith in and affection for their fellow man. They are dedicated physicians and scientists with a strong responsibility for the task fate has bestowed upon them.

Written in Cologne, Germany on the occasion of the 25th anniversary of the coining of the term pharmacokinetics by F. H. DOST.

Edward R. GARRETT, Ph. D. D. Sc.
Graduate Research Professor
College of Pharmacy
J. Hillis Miller Health Center
University of Florida
Gainesville, Florida

Foreword to the First German Edition

The authors of this work have been my collaborators for many years and have been particularly involved in practical aspects of pharmacokinetics. Our general interests have resulted in many invitations to give both introductory and postgraduate courses in pharmacokinetics, which have been generally intended for students with no prior knowledge of the subject but a desire to become acquainted with it.

The formulae and mathematical derivations on which our own work in this field is based are described in considerable detail in my book *Grundlagen der Pharmakokinetik;* they may at first sight appear rather complicated and forbidding to some biologists and medical people.

I therefore welcome the fact that Professors GLADTKE and von HATTINGBERG have been sufficiently motivated to give a written account of this course. It is intended as an introduction and also to orientate the reader in the subject. Some students will certainly be stimulated to study further this subject which I once called Pharmacokinetics (in 1953) without then realising that this term was to achieve worldwide usage in subsequent years. This little book will be a useful aid in their study.

Giessen, December 1972   F. H. DOST

Preface

The fundamental theory of pharmacokinetics has proven its extraordinary usefulness: It is now generally agreed that pharmacokinetic considerations provide the means to solve many problems in clinical pharmacology and that new drugs can be registered for use in man only if pertinent pharmacokinetic parameters are submitted by the producer.

It has become apparent far earlier than the founder of this discipline, F. H. DOST, ever attempted to predict that pharmacokinetics were accepted as an indispensable tool in medical, biologic, and pharmaceutic sciences.

Although the development of new approaches and methods in pharmacokinetics requires some knowledge of higher mathematics, they can be used and understood by the biologically oriented scientist and by the medical practitioner without advanced mathematical training.

Our text originated from introductory seminars. Unexpectedly, a second German edition had to follow after only 4 years. We have attempted to outline the basic concept of this relatively young discipline as simply and as comprehensibly as possible, and we have tried to avoid strictly mathematical derivations wherever this appeared permissible. Starting with the most simple definitions, we subsequently approached the more complicated reasonings and methods.

In two areas we gladly relied on the knowledge of two experts: Prof. Dr. W. KÜBLER wrote the chapter on pharmacokinetics in internal absorption, and Prof. Dr. W.-H. WAGNER compiled the section on the use of digital computer methodology. It was our aim to awaken interest in a new field and to prepare our readers for studying more specialized literature and periodicals recommended in the readings section at the end of the text.

We express our gratitude to the Springer Verlag for excellent technical quality, and we owe thanks to many members of its staff who provided helpful and important suggestions during the completion of this booklet.

Winter 1979   ERICH GLADTKE   H. MICHAEL VON HATTINGBERG

Contents

I. Volume of Distribution 1

II. Compartments 5
1. Protein Binding 6
2. Gastrointestinal Reabsorption 7

III. Elimination 9
1. Equation for Elimination 11
   a) Theoretical Initial Concentration 12
   b) Half-Time of Elimination 13
   c) Rate Constant of Elimination 16
   d) Total Clearance 16
   e) Saturation Kinetics 17
   f) Determination of Pharmacokinetic Data from Urine 20

IV. Steady State 22
1. Conditions for a Steady State 22
   a) The Exchangeable Pool 25
   b) Experimental Analysis of a Natural Steady State 26
   c) Endogenous Transfer 29
2. Artificial Steady State – Continous Infusion 30

V. Multicompartment Systems 35
1. The Model 35
   a) Invasion 37
   b) Concentration-Time Curve for Simultaneous Invasion and Elimination 38
   c) The Bateman Function 39
2. Dost's Principle of Corresponding Areas 43
   a) Test of Completeness of Invasion 45

    b) Rule of Corresponding Areas as a Supplement to the Basic Pharmacokinetic Experiment. 48
3. Dost's Rule of Corresponding Fractional Areas 50
    a) Fractional Quantities and Fractional Areas 50
    b) Conversion of Areas to Quantities of Substance 52
4. General Consideration of Multicompartment Models 53
    a) Multi-Exponential Function 54
    b) Subdivision into Individual e-Functions 55
    c) Practical Importance of the C; y-Expression. 57

VI. Pharmacokinetics and Treatment 62

1. Repeated Administration of a Drug. 63
    a) Duration of Accumulation. 63
    b) Degree of Accumulation 65

VII. Pharmacokinetics of Gastrointestinal Absorption 68

1. Gastrointestinal Absorption and the Bateman Function 68
2. Reconstruction of the Invasion Curves 72
3. Use of the Invasion Curves 74
4. Calculation of Dose-Proportional Absorption 78
5. Variants of the Invasion Process in Gastrointestinal Absorption 80
    a) Variants in the Site of Absorption 80
    b) Delay in Invasion Due to Lymphatic Transport of Lipid-Soluble Substances. 81
    c) Physical and Chemical Reactions After Absorption 82
    d) Excretion and Reabsorption of Substances in the Intestine. . 83
    e) Limitation of the Absorptive Capacity 84
    f) Different Absorptive Capacity of Two Segments of Intestine. 87
6. Conclusions 87
7. Appendix: Some Formulae and Their Derivation 88

VIII. Interaction 91

1. Elimination 91
    a) Pathological Changes in the Organ of Excretion 91
    b) Age-Dependent Changes in Elimination. 93
    c) Pharmacogenetic Factors 94
    d) Dependence of Rate of Elimination on Acid-Base Balance. . 94
    e) Circadian Rhythm of Excretion Rate 96
    f) Water Diuresis and Rate of Elimination. 96
    g) Solvent Deficiency 97

h) Enzyme Induction 97
i) Inhibition of Elimination by Toxicity 100
2. Volume of Distribution 102
   a) Hydration and Dehydration 102
   b) Hydropic States 103
3. Conclusions 103

IX. Use of Analogue Computers in Pharmacokinetics 104

1. Principle of the Analogue Computer 105
2. Programming the Analogue Computer 107
3. Use 110

X. Practical Application of Pharmacokinetic Procedures 115

1. Methods of Measurement 115
   a) Microbiological Methods 115
   b) Chemical Analysis 116
   c) Radioactively Labelled Substances 116
2. Assessment of the Results of Animal Experiments 117
3. Derivation of Pharmacokinetic Parameters and Constants . . . 117
   a) Calculation from a Graph 117
   b) Programmend Procedures 118
4. Mathematical Basis of Programming 118
   a) Distribution of a Substance Between Several Compartments . 118
   b) Blood Concentration-Time Curves for Pure Invasion 120
   c) Blood Concentration-Time Curves for Pure Elimination . . . 121
   d) Blood Concentration-Time Curves for Simultaneous Invasion
      and Elimination (Batemann Function) 122
   e) Accumulation, Limiting Curve 126
   f) Dosage Scheme 127
5. Examples of Calculation 127

Further Reading 137

Subject Index 139

I. Volume of Distribution

Every load with a drug, test substance or other material foreign to the body disturbs the natural steady state. The foreign substance enters the body by absorption from the gastrointestinal tract or an intramuscular or subcutaneous depot, by intravenous administration, or by some other route. In each case the substance appears in the blood, which simply acts as the organ of transport, although the lymph is sometimes an intermediate transport organ as well. The further distribution of the substance into other spaces is largely due to simple diffusion.

The volume in which the substance appears to be distributed behaves in many ways as a single enclosed space and may therefore be referred to as the central compartment. Compartments for further distribution, which are often more theoretical than actual, may be connected with the central compartment and with each other both in series and in parallel (Figs. 2 and 3).

The size of the volume of distribution which, in practice, is usually the central compartment only, is readily calculated from the principle of mixtures as illustrated in the following simple example.

If we empty a bottle of ink into a bucket full of water and stir well, the colour of the mixture is soon uniformly that of dilute ink. We can estimate the intensity of the colour roughly by eye or we can measure it precisely with a photometer. Clearly, the greater the quantity of water in the bucket, the paler the colour and the lower the concentration of dye. Hence the greater the volume of distribution, the smaller the concentration of the foreign substance, i.e. the two are inversely proportional to each other (Fig.1):

$$V \sim \frac{1}{y_0}$$

(V, volume of distribution; y_0, concentration of foreign substance)

This relationship may be inverted:

$$y_0 \sim \frac{1}{V}$$

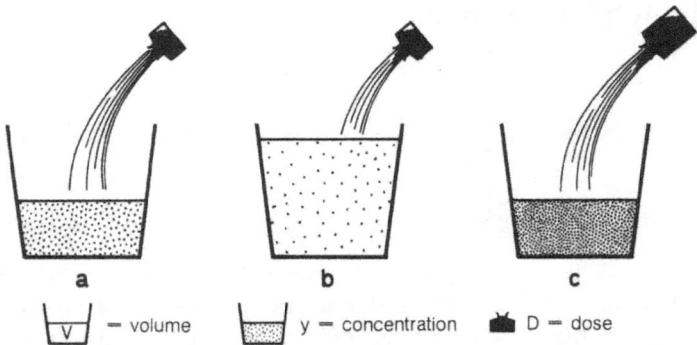

Fig. 1a–c. Concentration as a function of dose and volume of distribution.
a and **b:** When the same quantity of dye is added, the concentration in the vessel is inversely proportional to the amount of fluid present:
$$y \sim \frac{1}{V}$$

a and **c:** When different quantities of dye are added to the same volumes of fluid, the concentration is directly proportional to the quantity of dye added:
$$y \sim D$$

a, b and **c:** The concentration is directly proportional to the dose and inversely proportional to the size of the volume of distribution:
$$y = \frac{D}{V}$$

The dye concentration must obviously be greater when more dye is added, in direct proportion to the quantity added (Fig. 1):

$$y_0 \sim D$$
(D, dose)

These two proportional relationships are readily combined:

$$y_0 = \frac{D}{V} \tag{1}$$

This principle enables each value to be calculated when the other two are known, and may be applied not only to laboratory, household or kitchen equipment but also to the biological entity. The volume of a fluid such as plasma is measured by using a suitable test substance that is distributed solely in the space in question. An accurately known quantity of the substance is given and its concentration in the serum measured after thorough mixing. The two values, dose and concentration, give the volume of distribution and hence the size of the space in question, at least to a good approximation:

$$V = \frac{D}{y_0}$$

The extracellular fluid volume and the total body water may be measured similarly using other test substances. The intracellular fluid volume, for which we have no suitable indicator or measurement fluid at present, is then quite simply the difference between the total body water and the extracellular fluid volume:

$$ICF = TBW - ECF \qquad (2)$$

(*ICF*, intracellular fluid volume; *TBW*, total body water; *ECF*, extracellular fluid volume)

The estimation of these fluid spaces in healthy subjects and patients and particularly the detection of changes in their size due to different drugs is a major concern of clinical pharmacology. Changes in fluid spaces under the influence of diuretics, steroids, infusion fluids and nutrients of different mineral content give information about the activity of drugs and other effects.

Since, after administering a drug, the concentration of active substance in the blood and at the site of action depends, as shown above, not only on the dose but also on the volume of distribution, the size of the latter for the drug concerned must be known in order to be able to calculate dosage.

If we relate the volume of distribution of a substance to the body weight, we obtain the coefficient of distribution Δ':

$$\frac{V(\text{ml})}{BW(\text{g})} = \Delta' \left(\frac{\text{ml}}{\text{g}} \right) \qquad (BW, \text{ body weight}) \qquad (3)$$

We should stress that *for most substances, the volume and coefficient of distribution are theoretical quantities*. Several instances of coefficients of distribution greater than 1.0 are known, where the volume of distribution appears greater than the total volume of the body. This can only be explained by the loss of some of the substance in the equilibrium between the plasma and the volume of distribution, due for example to concentration by particular tissues or structures (e.g. by protein binding), to concentration in lipids or superficial structures, or to other processes. Some of the substance may migrate into deep or transcellular compartments (the eyeball, joint spaces, pleural cavities, effusions, cerebrospinal fluid), although the latter are seldom of quantitative importance except in special situations where they may indeed be critical for the effectiveness of a particular drug.

Only a few substances, such as antipyrine and ethanol, are distributed in the TBW. This distribution space is more or less proportional to the body weight. Many substances, however, are distributed in the ECF which is a laminar space of minimal height (the intercellular separation) and is therefore almost entirely determined by the extent of its surface. Its proportional relationship to the surface area of the body (BS) is proven experimentally:

$$ECF \sim 6.04 \cdot BS^{0.998}$$

The surface area is therefore a reliable guide to dosage in all age groups.

Finally, *the size of the distribution space for the same substance in the same person under the same conditions is always the same.* Changes in this distribution space indicate changes in the state of the body. Its size can be measured very reproducibly.

II. Compartments

The volume of distribution was described in the last chapter as a theoretical quantity. Strictly speaking, only the intravascular space is real. If, as occurs in diffusion, distribution is rapid and uniform, the volume of distribution often resembles a single compartment such as the extracellular fluid or TBW spaces. Where there are several distribution spaces, which incidentally need not conform with our pictorial image of a space, different effects are seen. If these spaces lie in parallel, as in Fig. 2, the solution is relatively simple.

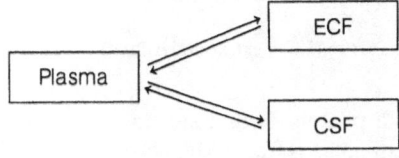

Fig. 2. Parallel compartments (*ECF*, extracellular fluid; *CSF*, cerebrospinal fluid)

Suppose the plasma contains a particular concentration of a substance which can diffuse from it into the extracellular fluid space. The concentrations in these two spaces (plasma and ECF) reach equilibrium. At the same time, the substance diffuses from the plasma into the cerebrospinal fluid (CSF), establishing another equilibrium. If there are no further changes and the compound is water — soluble and not protein — bound, then the concentrations in the plasma water, extracellular water and CSF ultimately become the same. Changes in the concentration in one space, for example the extracellular fluid, will react on the plasma and then the CSF concentrations. This model is simple to understand, easy to simulate with computers and quick to check and study simple by arithmetic operations.

1. Protein Binding

The relationships are somewhat more complex when several compartments are arranged in series. A very simple example is chosen here, for clarity (Fig. 3).

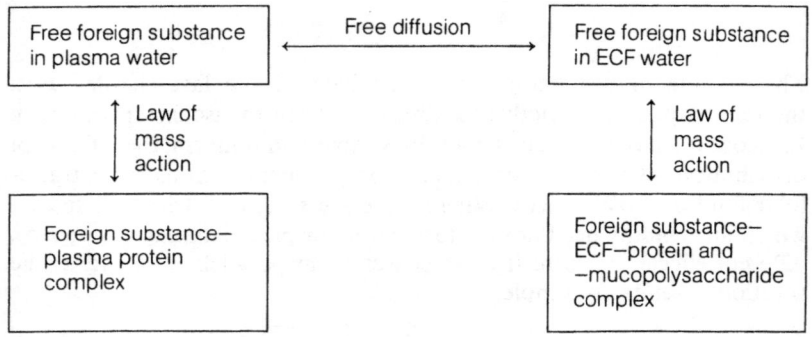

Fig. 3. Compartments in series (*ECF*, extracellular fluid)

Let us consider a protein-bound substance which is, therefore, partly unbound in the plasma, i.e. is free in the plasma water, and is partly bound to protein, i.e. forms a plasma protein–foreign substance complex. If the concentration in the plasma water rises, then so will the protein-bound fraction, and vice versa. This relationship obeys the law of mass action, and the Langmuir adsorption isotherms quoted for it can be derived simply from this law.

Some of this substance will obviously diffuse out of the plasma into the water of the extracellular space. This is a process of free diffusion which simply follows the concentration gradient. Proteins are also found in the ECF in concentrations of 0.5%–2%, and there are certainly other substances which will also bind the material introduced, such as mucopolysaccharides. Here, too, there is binding to protein or to some other substance according to the law of mass action or the Langmuir isotherm.

A marked change in concentration anywhere in this system will react, as indicated by the arrows in Fig. 3, on each of the other compartments. It goes without saying that smaller compartments or changes in the concentration of foreign material in them will have a proportionately lesser effect on the concentration in larger spaces. We may remind ourselves of the example of the ratio between the volumes of the aqueous humor and the plasma water.

Such interactions must nevertheless be considered even in compartments which differ greatly in size. An example of this is the fact that protein-bound substances such as the sulphonamides are normally found at very low concentration in CSF when compared with plasma. If we compare the concentration in plasma water with that in the CSF, however, we find identical values. The CSF of healthy people has a low protein content. If for any reason the CSF contains a larger quantity of protein as, for example, in inflammatory states, the protein-bound fraction of the sulphonamide will be considerably increased (Fig. 3), as will the total concentration in the CSF. In the very rare situation where CSF and serum have equal protein contents, they will also ultimately register the same total sulphonamide concentrations.

The 'better' penetration of many antimicrobial agents into the CSF when the meninges are inflamed is thus adequately explained. It is not better penetration into the CSF at all, but merely a displacement of the equilibrium by an increase within the compartment of protein-bound substance in the protein-containing CSF, and thus a rise in the total concentration.

Since antibacterial activity is associated predominantly or entirely with the non-protein-bound fraction of the antimicrobial agent, the effectiveness of an agent is not improved by this increased concentration in protein-rich CSF in inflammatory states, despite the regrettably numerous statements to the contrary. Such references are misleading and should not be made.

Improved perfusion or changes of membrane structure in inflammatory disease may nevertheless enable a substance to penetrate more readily into the CSF, possibly more rapidly than it can diffuse out again. Some studies with the cephalosporins and other antibiotics appear to support this observation.

Protein binding may often be disregarded when the same or approximately the same range of concentrations is investigated.

2. Gastrointestinal Reabsorption

The introduction of new, quite different types of compartments can also interfere with the calculation of concentrations and concentration curves. It was noticed recently that bromsulphalein is not eliminated exponentially, but that a smaller, second peak occurs towards the end of the phase of exponential elimination (Fig. 4). Suitable simulation with an analogue computer showed that gastrointestinal reabsorption introduces a new compartment which affects the course of the curve in this way.

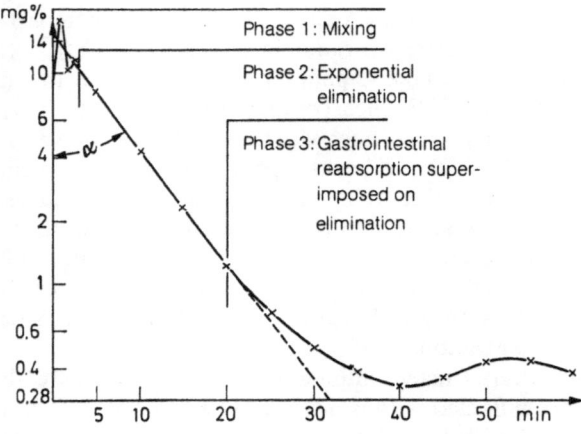

Fig. 4. The three phases of bromsulphalein elimination

A further example is doxycycline, a tetracycline distinguished by its long half-time of elimination (14–18h). The half-time is immediately reduced when intestinal reabsorption is inhibited, in this case to 4–6h, which is valid for all tetracyclines. Giving an iron preparation at the same time reveals this phenomenon, since chelates are formed which are virtually not reabsorbed, and this lack of reabsorption greatly accelerates the apparent elimination.

The circumstances described are clear and simple to interpret mathematically. We can show a similar phenomenon for para-aminohippuric acid (PAH). Here, more PAH is found in the intestine at the time of disruption of the curve and absorption takes place from this point onwards.

Models with 10 or more compartments are quite conceivable but, as a rule, only models with up to 3 compartments can be dealt with arithmetically. Models with more compartments than this must be pruned down until they fit these essential conditions.

If the biological importance and/or size of individual compartments differ greatly, most cases can be simplified by reducing the number of distribution spaces, whether they are in parallel or in series. One-, two- and three-compartment models are the simplest and are adequate in practice.

III. Elimination

Almost every foreign substance appearing in the blood and then the body tissues is ultimately eliminated, thereby restoring the original steady state. Elimination includes all the processes concerned in the removal of the substance in the form in which it was introduced or is observed from the compartment in question. This elimination can take place in many different ways, the most important of which are now reviewed.

A foreign substance can be excreted through the kidneys by glomerular filtration, tubular secretion, or both; it can be eliminated in the bile, either unchanged or after metabolism by the liver. Substances may be metabolised or catabolised in the liver, that is, broken down either completely or to substances normally present in the body.

These different routes of elimination are frequently linked in parallel or in series (Fig. 5). Moreover, when one route of elimination fails, another may be substituted for it or have greater demands made upon it. In severe liver failure, for example, the bulk, or at least a significant fraction, of the test substance bromsulphalein appears in the urine. Many other substances show a similar effect in liver failure or the reverse in renal failure.

All these elimination processes follow a law which can be expressed mathematically and described by relatively simple functions. The concentration in the blood generally falls in proportion to the concentration at

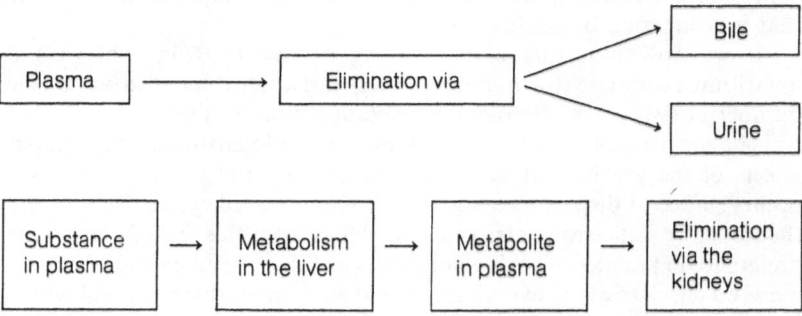

Fig. 5. Various routes and stages of elimination can be interconnected in parallel or in series

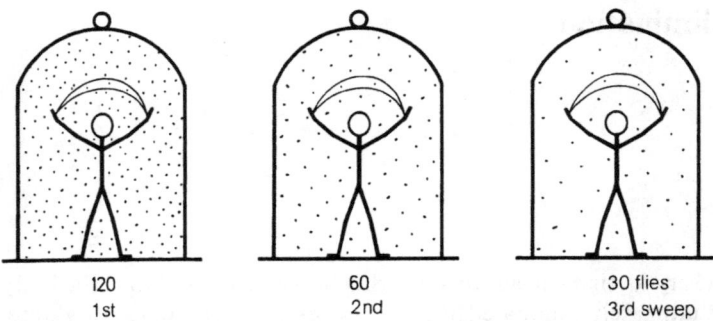

Fig. 6. Model to demonstrate elimination. Half the flies are eliminated at every sweep and so their number decreases in proportion, namely 120, 60, 30, etc

any given moment. This procedure may be clarified by a model (Fig. 6).

A man is standing in an enclosed space, illustrated here as a glass bell jar. A certain number of insects, for example flies, fly about in this space. The man has a net and, by a skilful movement, can catch some of them. Since the flies are uniformly distributed in the bell jar and he is able to free a definite fraction of the space of flies at each sweep of his net, he catches a certain percentage of them each time. Suppose that before the first sweep there are 120 flies in the container. The man catches half of them with his first sweep, leaving 60 with him in the space. These 60 flies are soon uniformly distributed again.

He now makes another sweep and again removes half the flies, that is, of 60 flies he catches 30. Equilibrium is then restored once more. With the next sweep he catches 15 flies, followed by 7.5. Each time, half the flies are removed, or eliminated. If we plot a graph of the number of flies on the ordinate and the sequence of sweeps of the net expressed, for example, as time, on the abscissa, we obtain the curve shown in Fig. 7 a. Even the least experienced mathematician will recognise this as an exponential function, that is, a function of the first order.

If we now plot this curve semilogarithmically (Fig. 7 b) with a logarithmic ordinate (the number of flies) and an arithmetic abscissa (the number of sweeps, or the time), we obtain a straight line.

The property of giving a straight line on semilogarithmic graph paper is one of the greatest advantages of an exponential function, and two points suffice to display this function. Two measured concentrations are theoretically sufficient to derive other values from this straight line. Our preference in practice of basing our curves on four to six measured points is merely a check to avoid experimental and analytical errors. We will return later to the advantages of this technique for expressing a curve as a straight line.

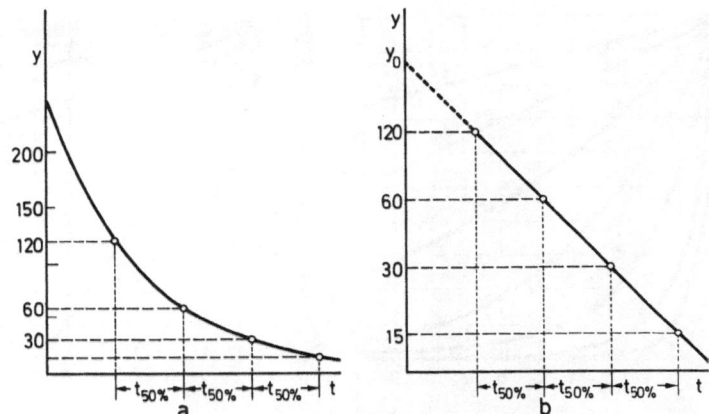

Fig. 7a. The model from Fig. 6, expressed as a linear plot. (Ordinate: number of flies. Abscissa: number of catches = time (t); $t_{50\%}$, half-time of elimination)

Fig. 7b. The same curve plotted semilogarithmically. The ordinate is logarithmic. $t_{50\%}$, half-time of elimination

1. Equation for Elimination

Some mathematical recapitulation is permissible here. The *decline* in concentration against time may be expressed as:

$$-\frac{dy}{dt} = k_2 y \tag{4}$$

This is a differential equation which can be integrated to give:

$$y = y_0 \cdot e^{-k_2 t} \tag{5}$$

Here, y is the concentration at any arbitrary time t; y_0 is the theoretical initial concentration at time $t = 0$; e is the base of the natural logarithm and k_2 the elimination constant, a value which will be explained in greater detail in section III. 1 b.

As already shown, this exponential function is expressed as a typical curve when plotted linearly and as a straight line when plotted semilogarithmically. A comparison of a series of curves in linear and semilogarithmic plots (Fig. 8) shows how much better the individual curves can be distinguished from one another when displayed semilogarithmically. Differences in the rate of elimination are much clearer and the half-time of elimination can be read directly from the semilogarithmic plot.

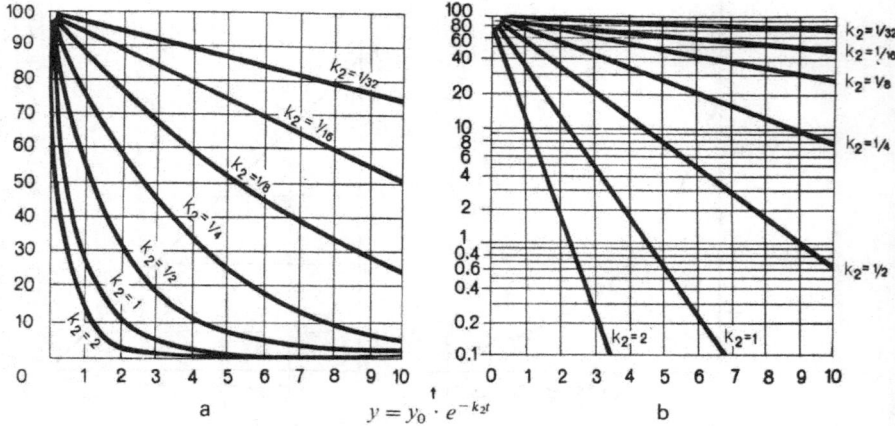

Fig. 8a and b. A number of curves plotted (**a**) linearly and (**b**) semilogarithmically. The rate constant of elimination k_2 gives the slope of each curve

The half-time of elimination is the time taken for the concentration to fall to one-half of its former value. It is of course the same for each segment of the straight line so we merely have to select a suitable segment. The procedure is shown in Fig. 8b and the difficulty of deriving the half-times of elimination from the same curves as linear plots is compared (Fig. 8a).

For clarity, we have so far deliberately considered situations in which invasion of the substance into the distribution space is very rapid in comparison with elimination, for example intravenous injection. We will continue with this assumption throughout the present chapter.

a) Theoretical Initial Concentration y_0

A further value of great importance for our calculations can be derived from the straight-line plots of elimination on semilogarithmic graph paper. By extrapolating the line in Fig. 7b back to its intercept with the ordinate ($t=0$), we obtain that concentration y_0 which would have been present at the time of injecting the test substance, had diffusion within the volume of distribution been instantaneous. This extrapolation of the concentration-time curve back to the starting time makes us independent of the continuous decline in the concentration of the substance under investigation.

The value of y_0, the theoretical initial concentration, must be known in order to calculate the volume and coefficient of distribution:

$$V = \frac{D}{y_0} \tag{1}$$

or else, with reference to the body weight,

$$\Delta' = \frac{D/BW}{y_0} \tag{3}$$

BW, body weight in kg

b) Half-Time of Elimination

In the differential equation, Eq. (4) and the exponential function, Eq. (5), derived from it by integration, a parameter occurred which we have called the rate constant of elimination (k_2). This value, which indicates the slope of the line in the semilogarithmic plot and is therefore a direct measure of the rate of elimination, is related to the half-time of elimination. The latter can be calculated from the rate constant of elimination. Conversely, the rate constant can be calculated from the half-time of elimination, as follows:

$$y = y_0 \cdot e^{-k_2 t} \tag{5}$$

$$\frac{y_0}{2} = y_0 \cdot e^{-k_2 t_{50\%}}$$

For the desired concentration y, we have substituted that concentration which is exactly one-half of the inital concentration y_0, i.e. $\frac{y_0}{2}$. Since, by definition, this concentration is only reached after one half-time of elimination has elapsed, t is equal in this case to the half-time of elimination. Division of the equation by y_0 gives

$$\frac{1}{2} = e^{-k_2 t_{50\%}},$$

making us thereby independent of the starting concentration.

Put into logarithms,

$$\ln \frac{1}{2} = -k_2 t_{50\%}$$

Reversing the signs,

$$-\ln \frac{1}{2} = k_2 t_{50\%}$$

Since $-\ln\frac{1}{2}=\ln 2$, we obtain

$$\ln 2 = k_2 t_{50\%}$$

By rearrangement,

$$t_{50\%} = \frac{\ln 2}{k_2} \tag{6a}$$

or $$k_2 = \frac{\ln 2}{t_{50\%}} \tag{6b}$$

The derivation of the half-time of elimination from the semilogarithmic straight-line plot of the concentration-time curve has proved to be extremely useful in practice. It forms the basis for the calculation of the rate constant of elimination. The rate constant of elimination and the theoretical initial concentration may equally well be determined from two measured concentrations:

$$\ln y_0 = \ln y_1 + |k_2| \cdot t_1 \tag{7}$$

$$k_2 = \frac{\ln y_2 - \ln y_1}{t_1 - t_2}$$

When there are more than two measurements, all the available information can be taken into account. Expression of the elimination Eq. (5) in logarithmic form gives the equation of a straight line:

$$\ln y = \ln y_0 + k_2 \cdot t \tag{8}$$

The usual arithmetic formulae for linear regression, in which the sum of the deviation of the measured points from this straight line is zero and the sum of the squares of the deviation is a minimum, may then be applied:

$$\ln y_0 = \frac{n \cdot \sum t_i^2 \cdot \sum \ln y_i - \sum t_i \cdot \sum t_i \cdot \ln y_i}{n \cdot \sum t_i^2 - (\sum t_i)^2} \tag{9}$$

$$k_2 = \frac{n \cdot \sum t_i \ln y_i - \sum t_i \cdot \sum \ln y_i}{n \cdot \sum t_i^2 - (\sum t_i)^2} \tag{10}$$

Thus, k_2 corresponds to the regression coefficient which is negative for a descending line. If the calculations in Eqs. (7) to (10) are performed by common or Briggsian logarithms (to the base 10), i.e. with log y_i instead of ln y_i, the right-hand side of the equation must then be multiplied by ln 10 = 2.3026.

The half-time of elimination is extremely important. We regard it as a standard value in biological metabolism, i.e. for the same substance in the same person under the same conditions, it is always the same.

Sulphonamides, for example, are classified on the basis of their rate of excretion into short-acting ($t_{50\%}$ up to 7 h), medium-acting ($t_{50\%}$ 7–16 h) and long-acting compounds ($t_{50\%}$ over 16 h).

There are comparably long-acting and slowly excreted tetracyclines which maintain an antimicrobially effective concentration over a long period on account of their prolonged half-time of elimination, and are therefore only given once a day.

'Depot' preparations, which also need to be given less frequently, depend on a different principle which will be discussed later. These compounds deliver their active component into the body in a retarded fashion with a resultant effect approaching that of continuous infusion.

Dosage calculations for the repeated administration of a drug, first worked out in detail by Krüger-Thiemer, are based on the half-time of elimination, which is directly related to the dose-interval, τ.

The half-time of elimination is also very suitable for function tests. It indicates how rapidly a substance is excreted and thus provides a quantitative estimate of the excretory function of the appropriate organ. Where a substance used, for example, to test renal function is eliminated more slowly, this indicates impairment of this function in the body.

Almost all the test substances known, such as bromsulphalein, PAH, inulin, thiosulphate, indocyanine green and many others, may be studied by the half-time method. The checking of dosage calculations also requires a knowledge of changes in the half-time of elimination of the drug concerned in relation to the norm so that the dose can be correctly adjusted.

The half-time method for function tests, introduced by Dost, has the great advantage that it is independent of the size, surface area and weight of the body. The measurements are therefore directly comparable with one another without further calculation, even when they are obtained from people of very different bodily dimensions. We have found this method to be particularly valuable in paediatrics and have made use of it for many years.

There is unfortunately *no such equivalence in the rate of elimination of the same substance by different species of animal.* Not only are shorter half-times regularly found for individual substances in certain animal species and longer half-times in others, but it has also not been possible to produce any coherent classification of these properties to date. *Calculations for drug dosage or function tests in animals must not be applied to man, nor vice versa.*

Our studies of drug dosage and clinical pharmacology have all had to be carried out in human subjects.

Interestingly, the Japanese authorities require all drugs to be retested in Japanese subjects even when they have already been thoroughly tested and used elsewhere. They obviously wish to protect themselves from unexpected variations in the pharmacokinetic and pharmacological properties in individual races. We are as yet unaware of any marked differences.

c) Rate Constant of Elimination

The rate constant of elimination k_2 is an expression of the extent to which a substance present in the volume of distribution is removed in unit time; $k_2 = 0.5$, for example, means that in unit time (e.g. 1 h) half of the substance is removed or eliminated. The rate constant of elimination k_2 is proportional to the reciprocal of the half-time of elimination, as already shown. Clearly, therefore, a value of 0.25 represents slower elimination than one of 0.5, whereas a value of 2 would mean more rapid elimination. Indeed, where $k = 2$, the substance could in theory be turned over twice in unit time.

d) Total Clearance

If we multiply k_2 (in hours^{-1} or minutes^{-1}) by the size of the volume of distribution (in millilitres), then we obtain a value whose dimension is millilitres/minute or millilitres/hour. This is that virtual plasma volume which is cleared of the substance concerned in unit time, and is the concept of total clearance. It embraces all the elimination processes in a single expression:

$$Cl_{tot} = k_2 \cdot V \tag{11}$$

For substances eliminated completely or almost completely by a particular organ such as the kidney or liver, total clearance is obviously the same as organ clearance. Thus the half-time of elimination of inulin or PAH, for example, enables us to calculate the renal clearance, and the half-time of elimination of bromsulphalein gives the hepatic clearance. In both cases, the half-time of elimination is converted into the rate constant $\left(k_2 = \dfrac{\ln 2}{t_{50\%}}\right)$ and then multiplied by the volume of distribution:

$$Cl_{tot} = \frac{\ln 2}{t_{50\%}} \cdot V \tag{12}$$

The dimensions must be standardised, e.g. to millilitres/minute.

e) Saturation Kinetics

(Non-linear pharmacokinetic systems)

Not all the mechanisms involved in the elimination of endogenous or foreign substances from the body strictly obey simple linear elimination kinetics or a first-order reaction. If elimination is mediated by enzymatic metabolism or by carrier-dependent transport systems in the appropriate organ, then the limiting capacity of such a system may become apparent as it can prevent the rate of elimination from increasing in proportion to the increasing dose. Instead, a maximal value is reached which is not then exceeded, despite further increases in dose. Such elimination kinetics may, like enzymatic reactions, be described mathematically using the Michaelis-Menten equation.

$$-\frac{dy}{dt} = \frac{V_m \cdot y}{K_m + y} \tag{13 a}$$

$-\frac{dy}{dt}$ is the rate of decline in the blood concentration after an intravenous injection at time t, and y is the blood concentration at time t. V_m, a virtual quantity in this equation, expresses the maximum total rate of elimination and K_m is by definition that blood concentration at which the rate of elimination is one-half the maximum possible.

These parameters enable those processes of elimination which obey saturation kinetics to be defined. An example is the elimination of the dye indocyanine green, which is rapidly distributed after intravenous injection within the intravascular space only, and is taken up selectively by the liver. Since the capacity of such hepatic uptake is limited, the rate of elimination changes as the dose of the dye increases, i.e. the apparent half-time of elimination is longer and the rate constant of elimination smaller (Fig. 9).

Since experimental conditions do not usually permit one to use as high a dosage as one would like in order to determine the maximum elimination capacity, the parameters characteristic of saturation kinetics must be calculated from submaximal dosage. Assuming a single-compartment model system, the initial rate of elimination V_0 is determined for doses of varying size. This is defined by the product of the rate constant of elimination k_2 and the theoretical starting concentration y_0 at time $t=0$. The equation $V_0 = y_0 \cdot k_2$ is obtained. If the rate of elimination at different

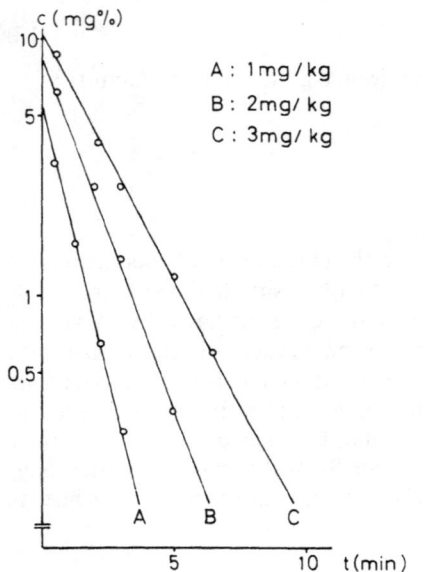

Fig. 9

doses is plotted against the dose given or, better, against the appropriate theoretical starting concentration y_0, the resulting curve tends asymptotically towards a maximum which is the maximal rate of elimination V_m (Fig. 10).

When displaying the characteristics of saturation kinetics graphically, it is helpful to modify the Michaelis-Menten equation according to Lineweaver and Burke by plotting the reciprocal value of the rate of

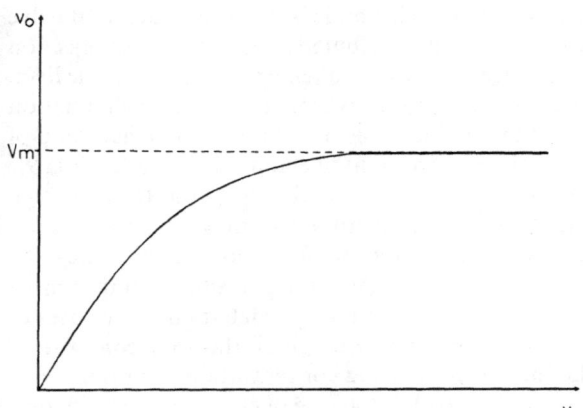

Fig. 10

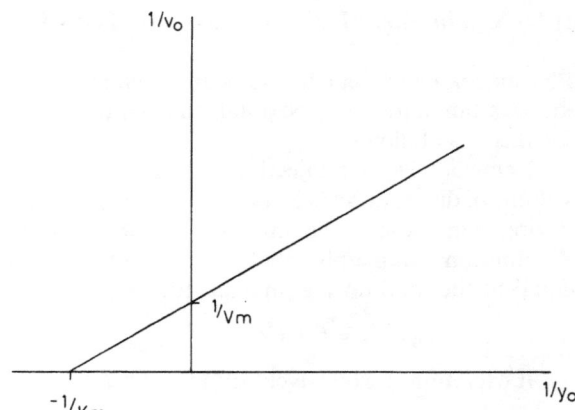

Fig. 11

elimination $\frac{1}{V_0}$ against the reciprocal of the theoretical plasma concentration $\frac{1}{y_0}$ (Fig. 11). This gives a straight line which intercepts the ordinate at $\frac{1}{V_m}$ and the abscissa at $-\frac{1}{K_m}$. These quantities can be read directly from the curve.

The fact that most drugs rarely show saturation kinetics at standard dosage is due to the fact that K_m usually exceeds the actual blood concentration y by a considerable margin. Equation (13 a) can then be reduced to:

$$-\frac{dy}{dt} = \left(\frac{V_m}{K_m}\right) \cdot y \qquad (13\,\text{b})$$

The similarity of this equation and that expressing first-order elimination (see p. 11) is obvious. $\frac{V_m}{K_m}$ in such cases is the same as the rate constant of elimination k_2.

A few substances such as ethanol and the salicylates, which may be taken in very high doses, can have a blood concentration y considerably in excess of K_m. In such cases the Michaelis-Menten equation can be reduced to:

$$-\frac{dy}{dt} = V_m \qquad (13\,\text{c})$$

This means, however, that elimination occurs at a constant rate independently of the concentration of the substances in the blood.

f) Determination of Pharmacokinetic Data from Urine

Pharmacokinetic data for substances eliminated quantitatively by the kidneys can quite easily be obtained from the urine. The theoretical basis for this is as follows:

Immediately after injecting a dose D_0, the absolute quantity in the volume of distribution is F_0 (assuming complete distribution). At any time during elimination, the amount of substance F still present in the distribution volume plus the quantity already excreted in the urine U is equal to the total dose administered:

$$D_0 = F_0 = F + U; \tag{14a}$$

If excretion is exclusively urinary,

$$F + U = U_\infty = D_0 \tag{14b}$$

Figure 12 shows the time course of elimination from the blood (I) and the cumulative excretion of the substance in the urine (II).

Curve I obeys the equation:

$$F = F_0 \cdot e^{-k_2 t} \tag{15}$$

and $\ln F = \ln F_0 - k_2 t$

Curve II:

$$U = U_\infty (1 - e^{-k_2 t}) \tag{16}$$

and $\ln(U_\infty - U) = \ln U_\infty - k_2 t$.

The method for determining the rate constant of elimination from urinary excretion is clear from Eq. (16).

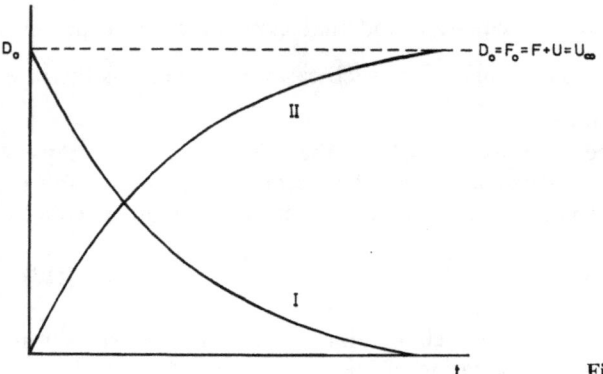

Fig. 12

The dose administered $D_0 = U_\infty$ is plotted semilogarithmically on the ordinate at time $t=0$. The urine is analysed, noting the time of stopping collection. The quantity of the substance excreted, U (concentration · urinary volume) is subtracted in each case from the initial dose $D_0 = U_\infty$. Thus the quantity $U_\infty - U$ remaining in the body is obtained and plotted logarithmically against time (on a linear scale). A declining straight line is obtained with a slope of $-k_2$.

IV. Steady State

1. Conditions for a Steady State

As explained in the previous chapter, most substances of exogenous and endogenous origin are eliminated at any given time and within certain concentration ranges at a rate proportional to their concentration at that time. This means that more substance will be excreted in unit time at high than at very low concentrations (Fig. 13). On the other hand, a substance can be introduced at a uniform rate into the distribution space, the compartment now under consideration.

If we introduce a substance by chronic intravenous infusion or if it passes endogenously from a particular organ or organ system into the blood, then the quantity of the substance entering this compartment in unit time will always be the same (Fig. 13).

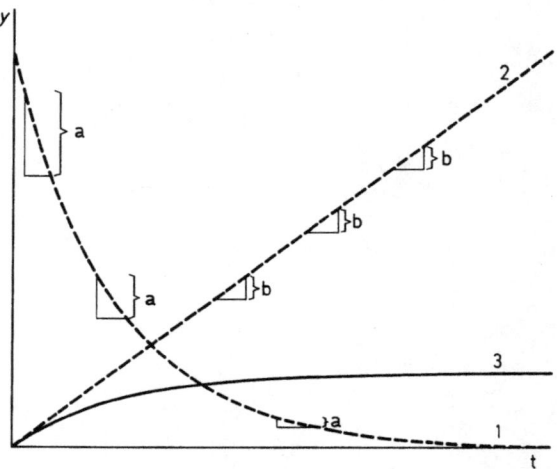

Fig. 13. Curve 1: Elimination. The quantity of substance, (a), eliminated in unit time depends on the concentration at that time. Curve 2: Inflow. The quantity of substance, (b), entering in unit time is always the same.
Curve 3: Steady state. Inflow plus elimination ultimately gives a steady state

If we now imagine both processes taking place simultaneously, then with intravenous infusion at a constant rate, only a small quantity of substance is removed in unit time at first, since the concentration is still low. The concentration rises, however, since input initially exceeds outflow. This rise is accompanied by an increase in the quantity of substance excreted in unit time until that point or concentration is inevitably reached at which the concentration excreted in unit time equals the amount delivered.

This process gives an ascending curve (Fig. 14), where the concentration eventually reaches a plateau. A steady state has been established in which the rates of input and outflow are the same. If we increase the rate of input, the concentration y^* in the steady state increases, whereas reducing the input makes this concentration smaller (Fig. 14 b–d).

There is therefore a direct relationship between the rate of inflow or rate of invasion v and the concentration in the steady state y^*. We can

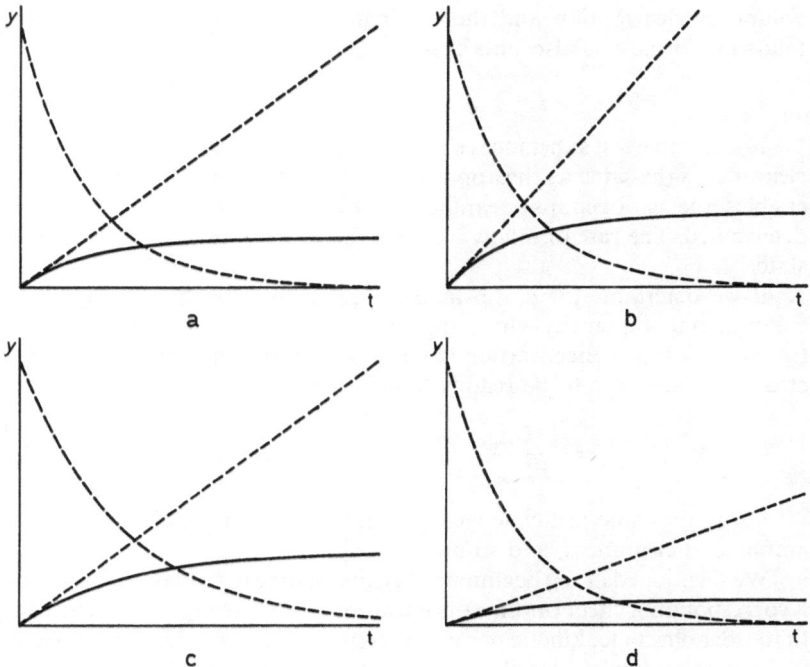

Fig. 14 a–d. An increased inflow (**b**) permits the concentration in the steady state to rise in the same way as a retarded outflow (**c**). A reduced inflow (**d**) or accelerated outflow, on the other hand, reduce the concentration

express this proportional relationship as a formal equation by introducing a constant:

$$v = y^* \cdot \text{const} \tag{17}$$

This constant is identical with the total clearance, as can be shown. From the above equation we obtain

$$v = y^* \cdot Cl_{tot} \tag{18}$$

If for v, the rate of in- or outflow, we substitute $U \cdot \dot{V}_u$, that is, the urinary concentration U, multiplied by the urine volume in unit time $\dot{V}_u$, and instead of y^* choose the symbol P for plasma concentration, we obtain the familiar formula for clearance:

$$Cl = \frac{U \cdot PV_u}{P} \tag{19}$$

Since, however, the total clearance is related to the product of the volume of distribution and the elimination constant ($Cl_{tot} = V \cdot k_2$), the following formula is also obtained:

$$v = y^* \cdot V \cdot k_2 \tag{20}$$

For suitable test substances eliminated by a single organ only, the total clearance is the same as the appropriate organ clearance. This procedure enables the endogenous clearance of a number of substances to be determined. The rate of inflow v equals the rate of outflow in the steady state.

If we determine for a substance excreted only by the kidneys (e.g. creatinine) that quantity which appears in the urine in unit time and also the steady-state concentration y^* in the blood, Eq. (20) enables the creatinine clearance to be readily found:

$$Cl = \frac{v}{y^*} = \frac{\dot{V}_u \cdot U_{creat}}{P_{creat}} \tag{21}$$

Using the same principle we can determine the urea, phosphate and amino acid clearances, and so on.

We mentioned at the beginning that any change in the rate of input has a corresponding effect on the concentration in the steady state, provided that other pharmacokinetic parameters remain the same. The steady-state concentration can be altered similarly by varying the rate of elimination. A delay in outflow causes the concentration y^* to increase just as does a more rapid inflow, whereas more rapid elimination results under otherwise identical conditions in a lower concentration. Many substances are present in the circulation under the sort of steady-state conditions just described, a fact which we often overlook when measuring and interpreting their concentrations in blood.

The body endeavours to maintain most substances at a uniform, constant concentration; sodium, potassium, calcium, phosphate, iron, amino acids, glucose etc. are examples of this. For other substances such as creatinine, urea or bilirubin, concentrations in excess of an upper limit or range usually indicate some pathological disorder of the in- and outflow equilibrium.

A change in the actual serum concentration of one of these substances, e.g. bilirubin, glucose or iron, is a sign of a disorder of the input-outflow equilibrium. An increase in the concentration can of course be due either to an increased inflow or to a reduced outflow.

Let us develop this argument further using bilirubin as our example. If the bilirubin concentration is markedly raised, the patient is jaundiced. One explanation for this is a raised inflow such as follows haemolysis and which is termed *haemolytic* jaundice.

The bilirubin concentration can also rise in a disorder of outflow from the blood. If hepatocellular uptake and coupling are disturbed, elimination from the blood is slower and the bilirubin concentration increases. For hepatitis and other forms of liver cell damage, we refer to *hepatocellular* jaundice. Accumulation in the liver cell resulting from mechanical outflow obstruction may also impair bilirubin excretion, causing *obstructive* jaundice.

These concepts also apply to other substances such as glucose and iron, for which a certain uniform concentration in the blood is recognised as normal. Suitable studies of the turnover of such substances in the blood give information about changes in the steady state, as will be considered in detail.

a) The Exchangeable Pool

When a substance is in steady state, that is, its input is the same as its outflow, a diffusion equilibrium must have been established within the volume of distribution. This would mean that a uniform steady-state concentration y^* must be present throughout the distribution space. Multiplication of y^* by the size of the volume of distribution is therefore a simple indication of the situation in the distribution space and is that quantity of substance which we call the readily exchangeable pool.

$$Pl = y^* \cdot V \text{ (mg)} \tag{22}$$

We can of course adjust this term for different body weights by substituting the volume of distribution for the distribution coefficient.

$$Pl = y^* \cdot \Delta' \text{ (mg/g)} \tag{23}$$

b) Experimental Analysis of a Natural Steady State

The question now is how to determine the volume or coefficient of distribution for substances which are normally present in the blood under equilibrium or steady-state conditions.

If we upset the steady state markedly for an endogenous substance by giving an accurately measured intravenous load of the same substance, then its concentration will rise above the steady-state level. Equilibrium is re-established by eliminating this disturbance.

The curve representing the disturbance of the steady state, in other words the curve showing the rise in concentration above the basal level (the initial concentration y^*), behaves as a simple concentration-time curve following an intravenous load (Fig. 15). It resembles an exponential function by approaching the initial concentration asymptotically in a similar manner to that seen with intravenous loading by an exogenous substance. The only difference is that, since endogenous material flows in continuously, the concentration prior to the experiment is not zero but an established starting or basal concentration y^*.

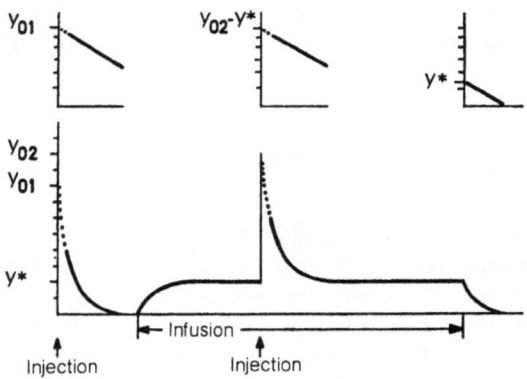

Fig. 15. Intravenous injection, intravenous injection during continuous infusion (steady state), and the concentration after discontinuing a continuous infusion all yield the same pharmacokinetic data (k_2, $t_{50\%}$, V)

This process may be illustrated simply both mathematically and experimentally and it thereby becomes clear that the same pharmacokinetic results are calculated from this disruption curve, i.e. the curve showing the elevation of the concentration above the basal value y^*, as from the time curve of the effects of loading with an exogenous substance. We performed a model experiment of this nature using PAH in such a way that a steady state was first achieved by continuous infusion at a constant rate (Fig. 15). Once a steady state had been established, an intravenous load was applied as a single injection of a suitable quantity of PAH, whilst the infusion continued throughout. The steady state was disrupted as can be seen in Fig. 15. Using this experimental model, for which a simple intravenous injection without a simultaneous continuous infusion was the preliminary stage, the half-time of elimination and other results could be obtained from all three portions of the concentration-time curve, namely the experiment before the continuous infusion, the intravenous load during the infusion and the curve after the infusion had been discontinued.

All three curves yielded the same half-time of elimination. Both intravenous loads gave an identical value for the volume of distribution as well as for the theoretical initial concentration. Thus an intravenous load with an exogenous substance enables us to determine the theoretical initial concentration, the volume and hence the coefficient of distribution, the half-time of elimination and the elimination constants. We must of course take great care not to insert the concentrations in our graphs or calculations until we have subtracted the value for y^*, the basal value, or the concentration in steady state. The information we require is only obtainable from the curve of elevation of concentration above the basal value.

In studies of sugar metabolism, this term is known as the glucose excess. Results comparable with those obtained from tracer experiments or in the absence of a steady state can only be obtained from this curve of concentration excess.

A different experimental concept may clarify this further. If we load the body with an exogenous substance, we obtain a series of concentrations which can be plotted graphically and which form the basis of our calculation (Fig. 16a). If for technical reasons any reagent or analytical blank values are found in the analysis, they must be subtracted before plotting the concentrations in order for the results to be comparable (Fig. 16b). In exactly the same way, the basal values must be subtracted before plotting the concentration-time curve, as is made clear in Fig. 16c.

An exponential function plotted semilogarithmically always gives a straight line, which declines in our case (elimination), i.e. it has a negative slope. If in plotting our graph we always add to each measured value a

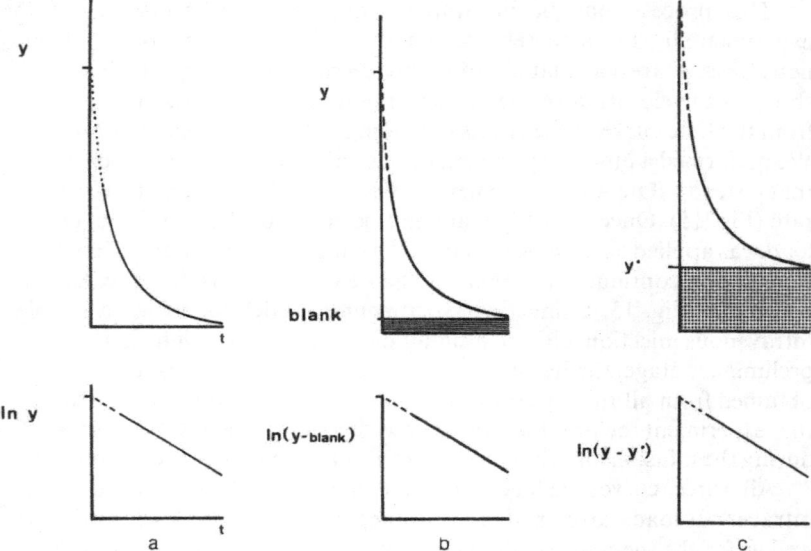

Fig. 16. a Intravenous load. **b** With analytical blank. **c** With a basal level ($y^{\cdot}$) in the healthy volunteer

fixed concentration or number, which is what the basal concentration is, then a new curve is obtained (Fig. 17). It is shown as the upper curve in this figure and is no longer a straight line, i.e. it no longer approximates to an exponential function, but is concave upwards. A similar but mirror-image curve is obtained when we subtract a fixed value from each concentration, as seen in the lower curve of Fig. 17.

If our concentrations lie on a straight line in this semilogarithmic plot, then our procedure is correct, for a logarithmically linear function is only possible when we have subtracted the actual asymptotes. If non-linear curves are obtained, this detail is the first which should be checked. Corrections for blank or basal values are unfortunately all too often overlooked.

One must of course also be prepared to check the correctness of the underlying model. The elimination curve for ethanol in man, for example, can never give a straight line on a semilogarithmic plot. Because of a deficiency in the degrading enzyme, ethanol is not degraded in proportion to its concentration but always at the same rate in unit time. Elimination is therefore a zero-order function and gives a straight line on a *linear* plot.

The elimination curve of a substance may, on the other hand, be affected over the period of observation by processes of both distribution

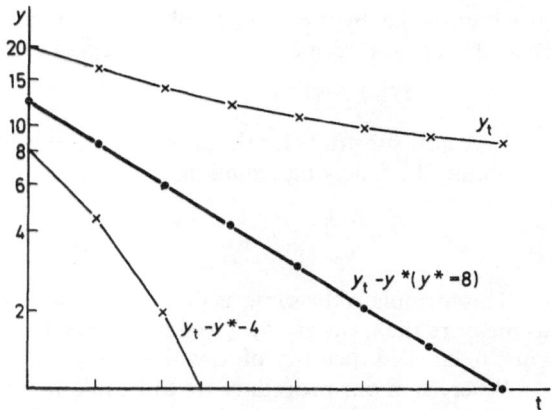

Fig. 17. Exponential function plotted semilogarithmically. Upper curve: basal level not subtracted, lower curve: overestimated basal level subtracted. Note resulting curvature

and excretion. The mathematical model for such a situation must take several compartments into account.

As previously explained, we can obtain the same information for each of these endogenous substances by intravenous loading with that substance and by suitable evaluation of the concentration-time curve, in exactly the same way as for an intravenous load of an exogenous substance. These indices are the half-time of elimination, the elimination constant, the volume and coefficient of distribution and the theoretical initial concentration which in this case is not y_0 but the elevation above the basal level, $y_0 - y^*$.

At the same time, we have learnt that the quantity of substance present in the volume of distribution may be determined simply by multiplying the basal value y^* by the size of the volume of distribution. This quantity in the distribution space is termed the readily exchangeable pool ($Pl = y^* \cdot V$ or $Pl = y^* \cdot \Delta'$).

c) Endogenous Transfer

We have also explained that the elimination constant k_2 gives information about that fraction of a substance contained in the volume of distribution which can be exchanged in unit time. It is therefore known not only as the rate constant of elimination but also as the turnover constant.

If this turnover constant is multiplied by the content of the volume of distribution, i.e. by the pool, we obtain the turnover in the blood in unit time. This is also termed transfer, as suggested by Dost.

$$Tf = k_2 \cdot Pl \tag{24}$$

If we now substitute for the pool the indices from which it is calculated, we obtain the following equation:

$$Tf = \frac{D \cdot k_2 \cdot y^*}{y_0 - y^*} \tag{25}$$

This formula is the same as that used in isotope and tracer techniques to measure the transfer of a given substance after the incorporation of a known, labelled quantity of it, which does not disrupt the equilibrium.

Whereas in our procedure we can confine ourselves to a single assay method of our choice which may be chemical or not, when tracer techniques are used to measure the rate of elimination and size of the volume of distribution, these same techniques must first be set up. The steady-state concentration y^*, on the other hand, has to be found by chemical analysis. The final calculation is identical and not only do the results obtained have the same significance but both methods actually also give the same values.

The endogenous turnover of many substances can be measured in this way. We can ascertain why the steady-state concentration is abnormally elevated or reduced and can also find out whether, for example, too much or too little substance is provided endogenously in comparison with the norm.

Turnover indices for glucose metabolism, bilirubin, phosphate and iron have been important to date, and it may be possible to study other substances by this method. The endogenous clearance of various substances can of course only be found because these substances obey the laws stated above.

2. Artificial Steady State—Continuous Infusion

The only situation so far considered is that resulting from a constant flow of a substance into the blood and extracirculatory distribution volume from an endogenous source, or exogenously in the form of an artificial continuous infusion. Such conditions initially offer the investigator an apparently static situation. The intrinsic dynamics of this system can only be demonstrated by some external disturbance such as an additional injection or the interruption of the infusion.

Continuous artificial infusion is occasionally performed for diagnostic or experimental purposes, since it permits the equilibrium of the sum of all compartments to be analysed. It is more commonly used, however, in the routine treatment of acute illnesses, enabling high or precisely known concentrations of a drug to be maintained over a long period. From this point of view, continuous intravenous infusion is the most reliable means of ensuring effective drug treatment. It is therefore appropriate to discuss the entire course of such concentration-time curves in greater detail.

If we understand the regular way in which, under conditions of continuous infusion, a substance tends to change its concentration from zero initially to a final, invariable, constant level, we can then assess its behaviour better and make practical rules for its intravenous infusion.

If, during a continuous infusion v (dose/time), a concentration equal to the steady-state concentration y^* in Eq. (20) arises, i.e.

$$y^* = \frac{v}{V \cdot k_2} \tag{26}$$

then this value remains constant throughout the remainder of the infusion, as shown by the interrupted horizontal line of Fig. 18. The concentration would otherwise decrease from its initial value y^* as

$$y_1 = y^* \cdot e^{-k_2 t} \tag{27}$$

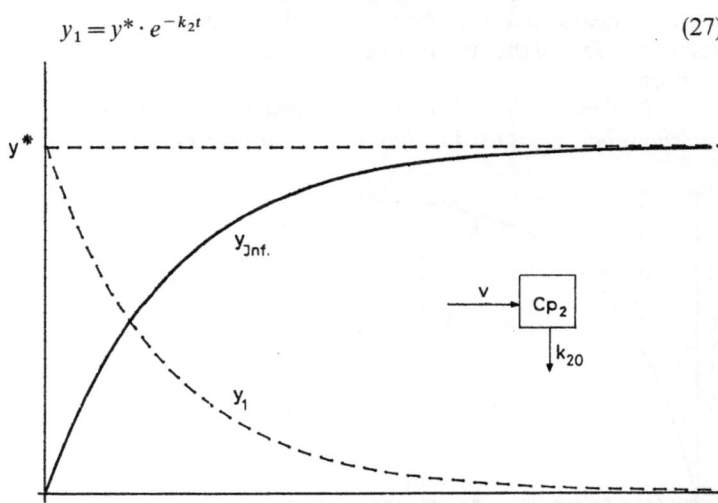

Fig. 18. Illustration of continuous intravenous infusion. *Interrupted horizontal line:* concentration curve during continuous infusion after a prior dose of $*D = y^* \cdot V$ y_1: concentration curve after a prior dose of $*D$ alone.
y_{Inf} concentration curve during continuous infusion alone, corresponding to $y^* - y_1$.
Ordinate: concentration

if there were no infusion.

The difference

$$y_{Inf} = y^* - y^* e^{-k_2 t} \tag{28}$$

therefore describes the concentration-time curve from the start of the infusion. The final form is derived with Eq. (26)

$$y_{Inf} = \frac{v}{V \cdot k_2}(1 - e^{-k_2 t}) \tag{29}$$

with an initial value $y=0$ and a limiting value $y^* = v/V k_2$. Note: this derivation is exactly the same as the integration of the differential equation for continuous infusion:

$$\frac{dy}{dt} = -k_2 y + \frac{v}{V} \quad |y_0 = 0 \tag{30}$$

The ascending part of the infusion curve should now be considered in exactly the same way as the elimination curve after a single intravenous dose. The half-time of elimination ($t_{50\%}$) here is that time in which the curve ascends by half of the difference between any given point and the asymptote (Fig. 19).

This means that after four elimination half-times, the concentration reaches 93.75% of that limiting value which can be achieved by continuous infusion.

A few important practical conclusions emerge: *if continuous intravenous infusion is used to determine clearance, an adequate time must be*

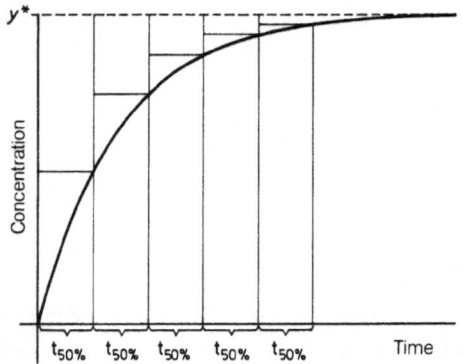

Fig. 19. Ascending part of a concentration-time curve during continuous intravenous infusion. Ordinate: concentration. Abscissa: time, marked with 'elimination half-times', for each of which the curve passes half the remaining distance to the asymptote

allowed between the start of the infusion and the collection of blood or urine. The usual procedures for calculating clearance assume that a steady- or equilibrium state has become established. Four to six elimination half-times are usually regarded as a safe interval before beginning the analysis in most cases. When this procedure is used for diagnostic purposes, the calculation must of course be based on the longest half-time that may be expected.

When continuous infusion is used therapeutically, on the other hand, the priority is not so much to establish a steady state as to achieve and maintain an adequate concentration rapidly. The time factor may be very important in such situations.

Chloramphenicol has a half-time of elimination in adults of about 4 h, so 16 h (= four half-times) must elapse before 93.75% of the final serum concentration is achieved, which would be a long period of inadequate therapy in a case of septicaemia. Penicillin G, with a half-time of elimination of 0.5 h, would reach a comparable concentration after 2 h.

This considerable practical delay in achieving active or equilibrium concentrations in the patient is easily avoided simply by giving a suitable priming or loading dose at the start of the continuous infusion, calculated in such a way that the concentration which would have been achieved by continuous infusion alone after theoretically infinite time is attained instantaneously at the start of treatment. The infusion then serves to maintain this concentration.

The requisite priming dose may easily and reliably be calculated from Eq. (20). For practical reasons, $\dfrac{\ln 2}{t_{50\%}}$ is substituted for k_2 and the half-time is expressed in hours.

Where the limiting concentration y^* is known, the priming dose ($^*D$) and the rate of infusion (v) may be estimated:

$$^*D\,[g] = y^* \cdot V \tag{31}$$

$$v\left[\frac{g}{h}\right] = y^* \cdot V \frac{\ln 2}{t_{50\%}} \tag{32}$$

If the aim is to maintain the activity of a single known dose ($^*D$) in this way, then the volume of distribution need not be known. The requisite maintenance rate v of the infusion is then

$$v = {^*D}\frac{\ln 2}{t_{50\%}} \tag{33}$$

Since $\ln 2 = 0.69 \approx 0.7$, *70% of the priming dose, divided by the half-time in hours, should be infused every hour.*

A common practice, particularly in chemotherapy, is to recommend a daily dose. This quantity, generally based on clinical experience, relieves the user of the necessity of calculating concentrations.

The rate of infusion is given as a dosage recommendation of d grams every 24 h. The priming dose $*D$ needed to achieve the limiting concentration y^* from the outset, is then

$$*D = \frac{d \cdot t_{50\%}}{24 \cdot \ln 2} = d \cdot t_{50\%} \frac{1}{24 \cdot 0.69} = 0.06 \cdot d \cdot t_{50\%} \tag{34}$$

Note that the size of y^* need not be known.

This means that *6% of the predicted 24-h dose should be given for each hour of elimination half-time if the full effect of a continuous infusion is to be achieved at the start.*

The rules derived from Eqs. (33) and (34) are very easy to remember and there is no reason why they cannot readily be applied to routine medical practice.

V. Multicompartment Systems

Pharmacokinetics is a means of quantitating the fate of a drug in the body. This means, more specifically, that all the mechanisms which the body brings to bear on a drug may be expressed in mathematical terms. The blood concentration-time curve is thus the result of a number of contributory processes to which the particular drug is subjected by the body.

When a drug is given intravenously, the rate at which it appears in the blood can be freely controlled by the investigator provided that he takes its pharmacological and biopharmaceutical properties into account; this rate is not, therefore, the expression of a biological process.

The intravenous route has the great advantage that the process of invasion can be ignored in the pharmacokinetic calculation. Rapid intravenous injection is therefore the basic pharmacokinetic experiment from which the important indices of the rate constant of elimination and volume of distribution are obtained. Continuous intravenous infusion can, moreover, yield additional information about very slow distribution and elimination processes.

Other modes of administration all have their own time relationships, however. The concentration-time curve always shows a delay and some of the drug may not even reach the circulation.

We shall now consider ways of analysing the time relationships and other quantitative aspects of various forms of drug administration, beginning with intramuscular injection, since the entire quantity injected can generally be assumed to pass into the blood via this route. This is important, since the blood concentration-time curve alone should give the necessary information, and only that quantity of substance which appears in the blood can be regarded as having been absorbed.

1. The Model

We assume, therefore, that the drug is deposited by injection into muscular interstitial tissue from which it enters the blood and is then distributed further into the extravascular compartments. Elimination takes place at the same time.

These conditions are illustrated most simply as a diagram (Fig. 20).

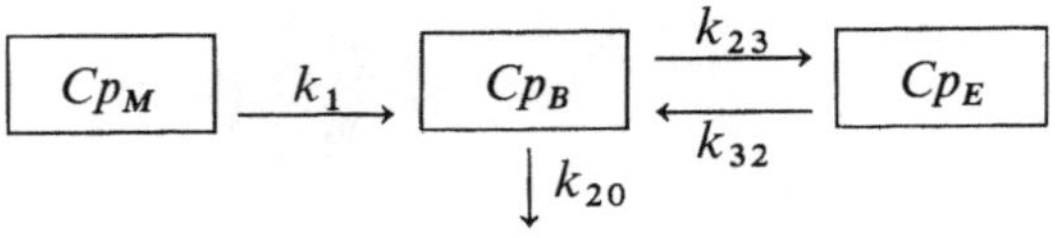

$$Cp_M \xrightarrow{k_1} Cp_B \underset{k_{32}}{\overset{k_{23}}{\rightleftarrows}} Cp_E$$
$$\downarrow k_{20}$$

Fig. 20. Diagram showing the basic pharmacokinetic model. See text for explanation

This figure, in which Cp_M is the intramuscular compartment of entry, Cp_B the blood compartment and Cp_E the extravascular compartment, which varies in size according to the substance, is the basic pharmacokinetic model. The coefficient k_{20} represents excretion and k_{23} and k_{32} are the rate constants of transfer of the substance between adjacent compartments.

The indices show the direction of the process: k_{23} (spoken 'k two three') is the coefficient of transfer from compartment Cp_2 into Cp_3; k_{20} represents transport from compartment 2 (blood) into an exit compartment Cp_0, which is not shown.

Where k_{23} is large in comparison with the elimination constant k_{20}, an equilibrium between Cp_B and Cp_E is soon established. The sum of the two then behaves as a single kinetic compartment Cp_2.

The simpler diagram of Fig. 21 is sufficient for most purposes. We will therefore restrict the following discussion to this more straightforward two-compartment model.

When converting a three- into a two-compartment system, it should be noted that the new elimination constant k_{20} is a single quantity made up of the original constants k_{20}, k_{23} and k_{32}. The influence of k_{20} and k_{32} therefore depends on their ratio to one another. In place of the blood compartment, there may be a central compartment with a volume larger than the intravascular space, but its kinetic behaviour as a transport organ is exactly the same as that of the blood.

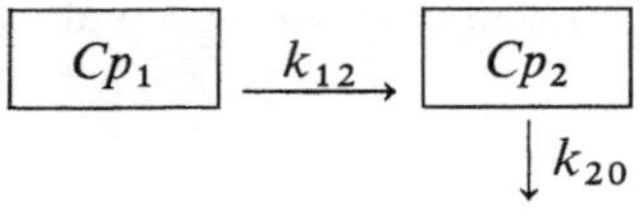

$$Cp_1 \xrightarrow{k_{12}} Cp_2$$
$$\downarrow k_{20}$$

Fig. 21. Simplified basic pharmacokinetic model. Cp_1 is the compartment into which the drug is administered and from which it invades Cp_2, the compartment where it is measured (the blood). This model corresponds to the Bateman function

a) Invasion

Invasion is the process by which a substance is transferred from the compartment of entry to that compartment from which blood samples may be drawn for analysis. Very complex interrelationships are involved for even the intramuscular injection of a soluble drug.

The pathway taken by a drug from its point of entry to its ultimate clearance from the blood may be subdivided into several separate stages, namely:

1) Diffusion within the solvent.
2) Diffusion through tissue and vascular membranes.
3) Transport by the blood.
4) a) Diffusion to the receptors responsible for pharmacological activity.
   b) Simultaneous diffusion into the fluid spaces accessible to the substance by virtue of its physicochemical properties. Together with the blood, these spaces are the most important components of the kinetically accessible distribution space.
   c) Diffusion to the organs of elimination.
5) Irreversible elimination.

Steps 1 and 2 can both be included in the term absorption. Subdivision into several steps is often necessary in biopharmaceutics, however, which studies the effects of galenic properties on kinetic processes. Thus the rate-determining step for oily depot preparations can be diffusion within the solvent, whereas the crystals of drugs given in crystalline form may form a separate initial compartment, so that the time course is governed by solubility in tissue water.

According to Dost, invasion is the sum of all these processes except for the fifth, elimination. The practical difficulty is that processes 1–5 all occur at the same time, so that elimination begins as soon as the first small amount of substance has entered the blood. Dost showed in 1953 that invasion may in practice be a uniform process which, like elimination, can display first-order kinetics.

For pharmacokinetic purposes, a *first-order reaction* is most simply described as follows: in the body, the particular substance is in opposition to a system which can remove a definite *proportion* of it as substrate in unit time. If the body always removes the same *amount* from the blood, as in the case of ethanol, the blood concentration of which can be of great medicolegal importance, then this is a pseudo-reaction of zero order, since the excretory enzymes in such a case are overloaded or saturated.

We assume that the substance deposited in the muscle leaves the site of administration at a rate proportional to its concentration there. We therefore proceed as in the derivation of the elimination equation. The rate of loss from the intramuscular depot is then:

$$\frac{dM}{dt} = -k_{12}M \tag{35}$$

If we stipulate that the quantity M_0 present at time $t=0$ is the same as the dose D given, then the equation is solved as:

$$M = M_0 e^{-k_{12}t} = D \cdot e^{-k_{12}t} \tag{36}$$

This equation shows how much of the substance M has still not left the depot at time t and so has not yet appeared in the blood. It has the same form as the equation describing elimination from the blood after intravenous dosage, Eq. (5).

That quantity B which has already passed into the blood at time t is then given as the difference:

$$\begin{aligned} B &= M_0 - M = D - M \\ B &= M_0(1 - e^{-k_{12}t}). \end{aligned} \tag{37}$$

The invasion curve which expresses the expected concentrations is then:

$$y_I = a(1 - e^{-k_{12}t}) \quad \text{with} \quad a = \frac{D}{V} \tag{38}$$

where V is the volume of distribution.

Since elimination occurs simultaneously, neither this curve nor the invasion constant k_{12}, which has been shown to differ from the absorption constant by including distribution and other processes, can be obtained directly from this experiment.

Dost and Kübler have each independently developed a method for determining these constants indirectly, as will be described later.

b) Concentration-Time Curve for Simultaneous Invasion and Elimination

We now have the task of describing the blood concentration-time curve for simultaneous invasion and elimination. Returning to Fig. 21, let us first write down the rates of loss of the quantities M and B from the muscle and blood compartments, that is, Cp_1 and Cp_2.

$$\frac{dM}{dt} = -k_{12}M \qquad M_0 = D \tag{35}$$

$$\frac{dB}{dt} = +k_{12}M - k_{20}B \qquad B_0 = 0 \tag{39}$$

Solving this system of differential equations, we obtain

$$y = a \frac{k_{12}}{k_{12} - k_{20}} (e^{-k_{20}t} - e^{-k_{12}t}) \tag{40}$$

where
$$a = \frac{D}{V} = \frac{M_0}{V}$$

The quantity a is exactly the same as the theoretical initial concentration y_0, which can be obtained by extrapolation when the same dose is given intravenously. It signifies either the dose as related to the volume of distribution V, or else the concentration which would be found if the entire dose were to be distributed immediately throughout the active volume of distribution.

c) The Bateman Function

Equation (40) was evolved in 1910 by Bateman and has been named after him (the Bateman function). It describes in mathematical terms the decay of a radioactive mother substance into another radioactive daughter substance which has its own half-life.

Since a few short-lived radioactive tracer elements used in nuclear medicine may be 'milked off' in the laboratory as products of the decay of a long-lived mother substance, this equation has some practical value for medicine in its original context also.

We see here the importance of *analogy*, which is frequently used in mathematics. The mathematical expression of two analogous processes, in this case pharmacokinetics and radioactive decay, is identical. The constant k, which describes a function of the body, and the decay constant λ, which gives the probability of decay of an atom, are analogous. The equation for the Bateman function is relatively simple in fact, but less obvious. It is therefore shown graphically in Figs. 22 and 23.

Curve I expresses a simple elimination function after intravenous administration and corresponds to Eq. (5). Curve II is the invasion curve which is a theoretical function in clinical pharmacology, since it cannot be obtained directly. Curve III is the curve obtained experimentally for a substance which leaves the site of administration at a rate proportional to its concentration there, and enters the blood where it immediately encounters the mechanisms of elimination.

Figures 22 and 23 differ purely in the fact that the ratio of the rate constants, k_{12} and k_{20}, is reversed. In Fig. 22, invasion is twice as rapid as elimination whereas in Fig. 23, invasion and elimination are in the ratio

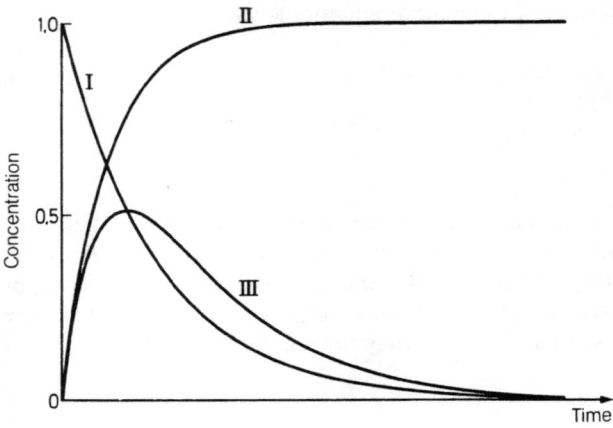

Fig. 22. The Bateman function plotted linearly. *I*, pure elimination (i.v. dosage); *II*, pure invasion; *III*, concentration-time curve for simultaneous invasion and elimination. $k_{12} : k_{20} = 2 : 1$. Ordinate: concentration in blood. Abscissa: time

1:2. Complete transfer of the same dose into the blood is assumed for all the curves and so *a* is the same for all equations. The flatness of curve III may therefore seem surprising at first sight.

Semilogarithmic Expression of the Bateman Function

There are some special considerations when the Bateman function is expressed semilogarithmically. The curve rises from minus infinity and

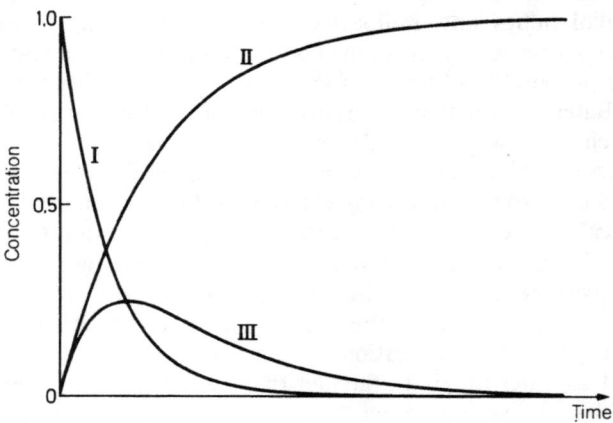

Fig. 23. As Fig. 22, except that $k_{12} : k_{20} = 1 : 2$

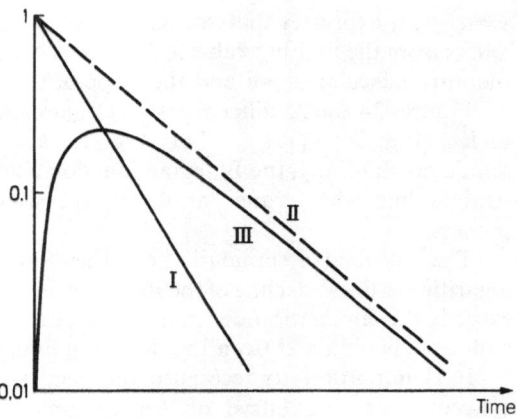

Fig. 24. Bateman function plotted semilogarithmically. *I*, pure elimination after i.v. administration. *II*, inverted invasion curve [from Eq. (36)]. *III*, concentration-time curve of simultaneous invasion and elimination. $k_{12} : k_{20} = 2 : 1$. Ordinate: concentration on a logarithmic scale. Abscissa: time, on a linear scale

passes through a maximum which lies by definition on the elimination curve after intravenous administration of the same dose. The curve then approximates to a declining straight line.

Figures 24 and 25 show the concentration-time course after intravenous (I) and intramuscular (III) dosage, with the concentration plotted logarithmically on the ordinate. The interrupted line (II) is an inverted logarithmic plot of the pure invasion curve. Through the function

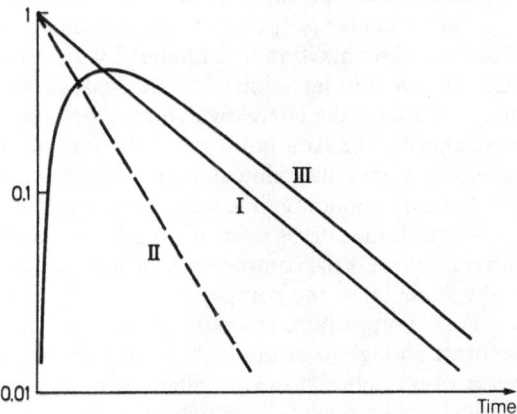

Fig. 25. As Fig. 24 except that $k_{12} : k_{20} = 1 : 2$. Explanation in text

$y = a - y_I$ it expresses that concentration by which the invasion curve y_I differs from the limiting value a. Thus the curve describes the emptying of the intramuscular depot and the slope of this line is determined by k_{12}.

Figures 24 and 25 differ exactly as Figures 22 and 23 by the ratio of k_{12} to k_{20} (Fig. 24: $k_{12}:k_{20} = 2:1$; Fig. 25: $k_{12}:k_{20} = 1:2$). When plotted semilogarithmically, the Bateman function changes asymptotically into a straight line which runs parallel to the slower corresponding partial process.

The half-time of elimination can therefore only be obtained from the logarithmic-linear decline of the Bateman function if the invasion constant exceeds the elimination constant. When the reverse is true, an 'invasion half-time' is obtained from the declining limb of the curve!

It is important to recognise this fact, since analysis of the blood concentration-time curve of, for example, intramuscular benzathine penicillin or iron, or of oral preparations of substances such as iron, which are slowly and hence often incompletely absorbed, can falsify the estimation of the elimination half-time.

Figures 24 and 25 also show that one cannot obtain y_0 by extrapolating the declining part of the curve back to the ordinate.

The theoretical initial concentration y_0 or a may be determined by graphic extrapolation when k_{12} is greater than k_{20} and when the maximum value of the curve is sufficiently exactly known. The curve for pure elimination may then be reconstructed by a parallel displacement of the declining phase to pass through the maximum. This procedure is of general practical application, since k_{12} for most drugs other than depot preparations is considerably larger than k_{20}. Where $k_{12} = k_{20}$, this principle cannot be applied, since the curve is not then a straight line.

The particular properties of the Bateman function have already been described. The maximum value lies by definition on the curve obtained after intravenous injection of the same dose, as is clear from Fig. 26. This diagram shows the curves which may be expected for different invasion constants but the same half-time of elimination. The dose is the same for all curves. It is obviously almost impossible to determine the maximum value and the corresponding time with sufficient accuracy when the curve is flat.

Since all the curves refer to the same dose, the height of the maximum can only express the completeness of invasion where the invasion constant is the same in all the comparisons.

This is important, since the concept of the Bateman function is still accurate enough to be applied to many aspects of enteric absorption. The restriction applies, however, when several compartments are invaded in parallel or in sequence, in which cases the peak concentration again gives no indication of the completeness of invasion.

2. Dost's Principle of Corresponding Areas

Our discussions so far have shown that the concentration of a drug in the blood at any time appears to depend on at least four quantities. These are the dose taken up into the volume of distribution, the size of the volume of distribution, the rate constant of elimination and the rate of invasion, which is defined for the Bateman function by a single rate constant and for other cases by several constants. Since the volume of distribution and the elimination constants of a substance are standard biological quantities for the individual person and remain constant except for biological variation, considerable simplification is possible, as follows. The area under each curve in Fig. 26 is the same, namely

$$S = \frac{a}{k_{20}} = \frac{D}{V \cdot k_{20}} = \frac{D}{Cl_{tot}} \left[\frac{mg \cdot h}{ml} \right] \tag{41}$$

In determining this area mathematically as the integral of Eq. (40), the indices associated with invasion disappear. The area S then depends only on the total dose appearing in the blood and the total clearance Cl_{tot}.

Equation (41) is the mathematical expression of the Rule of Corresponding Areas in pharmacokinetics, first recognised by Dost. It is often referred to as Dost's Principle and may be demonstrated as follows.

Figure 27 illustrates a simple concept: if two different doses of a substance enter the circulation by any route (the same for both), then the

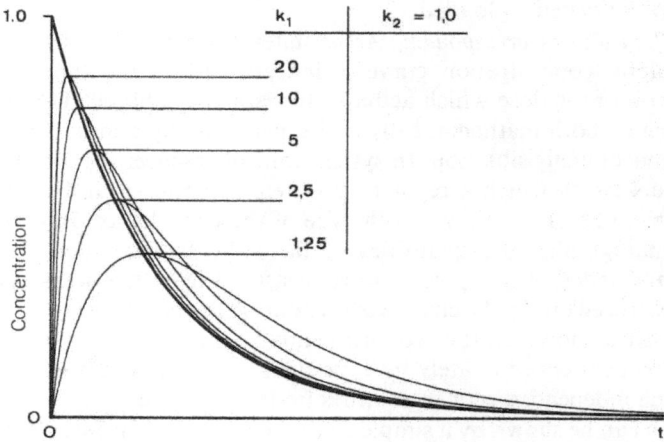

Fig. 26. The Bateman function when k_{12} varies and k_{20} remains constant. All the maxima lie on the curve given by $k_{12} = \infty$ (rapid intravenous administration) of the same dose. The areas under all the individual curves are the same. Ordinate: concentration. Abscissa: time

43

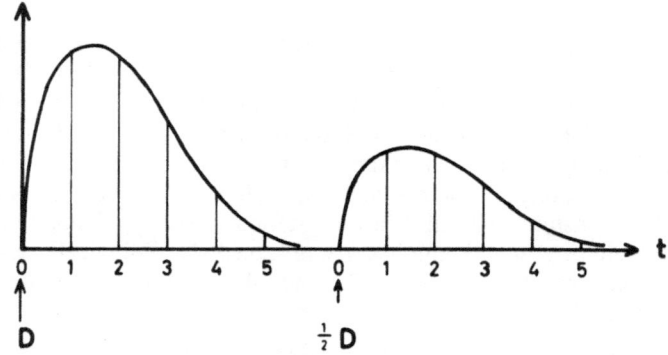

Fig. 27. Concentration-time curves for the same (intramuscular) administration of different doses of the same drug. Concentrations at comparable times of measurement are in the ratio of the doses administered (1 : 0.5). Ordinate: concentration. Abscissa: time

blood concentrations at comparable times after administration are in the ratio of the doses, i.e. are dose proportional. The same also applies to the product of these concentrations with comparable time intervals.

If the time axis is now divided into very small segments, the sum of the products of these segments with their corresponding concentrations is equal to the area under the concentration curve. Thus the total area under the concentration curve is proportional to the quantity of substance with which the system is loaded.

The Rule of Corresponding Areas states in general that the area under the blood concentration curve is independent of the time course of invasion of the dose which actually appears in the blood. This has been confirmed both mathematically and experimentally and is not a special pharmacokinetic situation. In system control engineering, the integral of the curve with which a regulatory system responds to a disturbance is known to be proportional to the size of the disturbance. In all types of chromatography, the quantities of the individual components of the mixture undergoing separation are measured from the areas under the curves traced out by the chart recorder during the process of separation. In many cases, however, the proportionality factor has to be determined for each component separately by constructing standard curves.

The independence of these areas from the form and rate of administration can be shown by a simple clinical experiment. In Fig. 28, the same dose of PAH was injected intravenously both rapidly and at different infusion rates. The three curves have different forms but the areas under them are all the same.

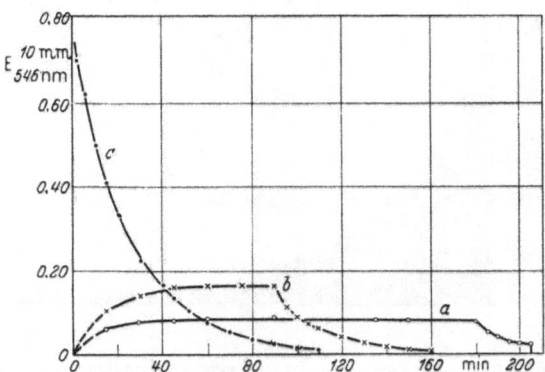

Fig. 28. Concentration-time curves of PAH in the same volunteer during and after 22.6 mg/kg, i.v. *a* Continuous infusion for 180 min. *b* Continuous infusion for 90 min. *c* Single rapid injection. The areas under all the curves are the same. Ordinate: concentration, expressed as the extinction value of the measurement system of a photometer at 546 nm and 10-mm layer thickness. Abscissa: time in minutes

a) Test of Completeness of Invasion

Since dose and area are proportional, the completeness of invasion may be determined quantitatively after any desired route of administration. If the same drug is given on two separate occasions, each time by a different route (e.g. by intravenous injection, where invasion is by definition complete, and by mouth), then the measure of agreement between the areas obtained is an index of the completeness of absorption by the latter route.

Since S is the integral of the blood concentration curve between zero and infinity, the total area must be measured. The blood concentration-time curve has to be followed until it no longer differs from zero. If the last chemically estimated concentration still shows a significant value, the remaining part of the area can be obtained from Eq. (41) by substituting this value for a.

In practice, very little computation is required when determining the completeness of enteric invasion experimentally. The values y_0, V and k_{20} are first determined in the usual way by the rapid intravenous infusion of a precisely measured dose, D_{iv}. The area S_{iv} corresponding to the dose D_{iv} (Fig. 29) is then given by Eq. (41).

A second known dose, D_{app}, is then given by the route under investigation, e.g. by rectal suppository. The resulting blood concentration-time curve is now followed by frequent analysis over the time during which absorption is to be assessed (Fig. 30).

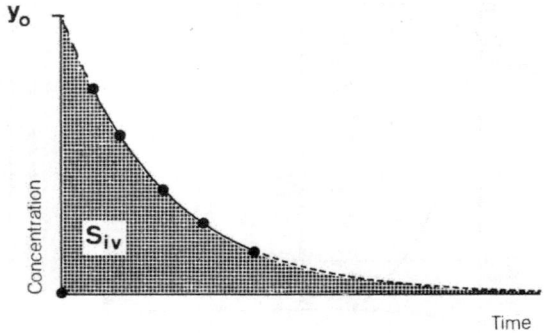

Fig. 29. Corresponding areas after intravenous administration of a known dose. $S_{iv} = y_0/k_{20}$. Ordinate: concentration. Abscissa: time, on the same scale as that to which k_{20} relates

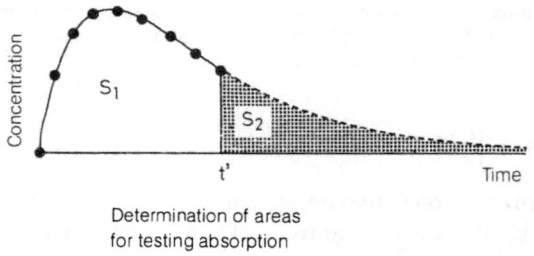

Determination of areas
for testing absorption

Fig. 30. Corresponding areas of the absorbed portion of a dose given by any desired route. $S_{abs} = S_1 + S_2 = S_1 + y_{t'}/k_{20}$. S_1 is determined pragmatically. Ordinate: concentration. Abscissa: time

The area designated S_1 in Fig. 30 is measured pragmatically. This is done either by means of a polar planimeter or mathematically by use of the trapezoid formula.

$$S_1 = \sum_{t_0}^{t'} \frac{y_{n-1} + y_n}{2} (t_n - t_{n-1}) \tag{42}$$

Another simple method is to plot the curve on graph paper, cut it out with scissors and weigh the cut-out on an analytical balance. In this procedure the weight must be converted to the same dimension $\left(\dfrac{g \cdot h}{ml}\right)$ as is used in Eq. (41) and (42).

The area S_1 determined by each of the above methods between t_0 and t' is related to the amount of substance which has entered the blood up to time $t = t'$ and has then left it again. This quantity is termed *transit*.

The area S_2, which corresponds to the amount of drug still present in the blood at time $t=t'$, on the other hand, is given by

$$S_2 = \frac{y_{t'}}{k_{20}} \tag{43}$$

The area which corresponds to the dose D_{abs} absorbed into the blood from the site of administration up to time t' is then the sum of both partial areas.

$$S_{abs} = S_1 + S_2 \tag{44}$$

The proportion of the dose D_{app} given in the second experiment and actually absorbed is equal to the ratio of the areas $S_{abs}:S_{iv}$, taking the actual doses given, which need not be the same, into account.

$$\frac{D_{abs}}{D_{app}} = \frac{S_{abs}}{S_{iv}} \cdot \frac{D_{iv}}{D_{app}} \tag{45}$$

Evaluating the absorption of a drug can therefore be reduced to a comparison of two areas, which requires little mathematical effort, or even to the simple comparison of the weights of two pieces of paper. All that is required is a series of measured concentrations in the blood or serum.

Practical Example

Using this principle, phenylbutazone was found to be almost completely absorbed after oral administration but only about one-half was absorbed when given rectally, using two different preparations (Table 1). This means that the doctor must give twice the dose by suppositories or rectal capsules to achieve the same concentrations as are found after taking the oral preparation.

Table 1. The enteric absorption of phenylbutazone

Route	No.	Absorption (% of dose)
Oral	5	84.2 ± 21
Rectal (phenylbutazone)	11	54.0 ± 21
Rectal (proprietary preparation of phenylbutazone, heptobarbitone and amidopyrine as rectal capsules)	15	47.3 ± 25

The dose necessary for the rectal administration of a potent antipyretic analgesic of this nature can also be titrated clinically, on the basis of relief of symptoms, with fair reliability. The effect can be recognised by the

Table 2. Percentage absorption after giving sulphonamides orally and rectally

Sulphonamide	Oral		Rectal		No.
	Mean %	Standard deviation	Mean %	Standard deviation	
Sulphaethylpyrimidine	101.5		–	–	–
Sulphisomidine	98.3	9.3	30.0	8.6	7
Sulphadimethyloxazole	90.3		39.0	7.3	6
Sulphamethoxydiazine	98.6	$n = 29$	18.0	6.1	8
Sulphadimethoxine	94.5	$(v = 24)$	39.0	17.3	6
Sulphafurazole	–		49.0	16.2	6

doctor after a short period so that the dose can be gradually increased in the individual case until the desired effect is achieved.

Other considerations apply to drugs whose activity depends on their concentration not falling below a certain minimum over a long period of time, such as the antimicrobial agents.

Table 2 summarises the absorption properties of sulphonamides for oral and rectal use. Absorption after oral dosing is almost complete for all the drugs studied and the standard deviation, a measure of the reliability of the information, is 9.3%.

Important differences are seen with the rectal route. The percentage of sulphamethoxydiazine is clearly below that of the other compounds. Experience with one sulphonamide cannot therefore necessarily be applied to others.

More importantly, there is a considerable difference in the reliability of the rectal route for different sulphonamides. The standard deviations in the rectal absorption of sulphadimethoxine and sulphafurazole are considerably greater than those for the other preparations. Reliable therapy is not ensured by considering the mean absorption loss alone.

We conclude that it is unsafe to use a suppository as the galenic formulation of any substances which show a delay in the onset of their effects sufficient to prevent the reliable adjustment of their dosage on clinical grounds. Uncontrolled, ineffective therapy with potent agents is dangerous and runs the risk of side-effects such as allergy.

b) Rule of Corresponding Areas as a Supplement to the Basic Pharmacokinetic Experiment

The results of the half-time of elimination and volume of distribution as determined by the basic pharmacokinetic experiment of rapid intravenous infusion are sometimes difficult to check.

Such difficulties are to be expected when distribution is much slower than elimination, so that equilibration does not occur within the volume of distribution during the period of the experiment. The increase in volume of distribution with increasing dose must be taken into account here, since more drug can penetrate the less accessible compartments at high concentrations.

To exclude this effect, a precise quantity of the drug can be infused so slowly that the desired equilibrium is set up in all compartments. The infusion does not need to be at a uniform rate. The total area under the concentration curve from the start of the infusion to complete elimination from the blood then corresponds to the dose infused. Since all attainable compartments are in equilibrium at the end of the infusion, the elimination curve soon assumes a logarithmic-linear course in a period when it can still be analysed. The effective half-time of elimination for the entire volume of distribution can be determined from this and its size calculated from Eq. (41).

The same process may be used to determine the pharmacokinetic parameters for substances which, for galenic reasons, are unsuitable for rapid injection in the requisite dose, or where the peaks of concentration found before distribution cause toxicity or have unpleasant effects. The ratio between dose and area is the same as that between the rate of infusion and the concentration y^* in the steady state during continuous intravenous infusion:

$$\frac{D\,[\text{mg}]}{S\,[\text{mg}\cdot\text{ml}^{-1}\cdot\text{h}]} = \frac{v\,[\text{mg}\,\text{h}^{-1}]}{y^*\,[\text{mg}\,\text{ml}^{-1}]} = V\,[\text{ml}]\cdot k_{20}\,[\text{h}^{-1}] = Cl_{tot}\,[\text{ml}\,\text{h}^{-1}] \quad (46)$$

Which of the two possible procedures is preferred is solely an organisational and technical question. A continuous infusion may be difficult to maintain for long periods with the necessary accuracy and uniformity of rate. Conversely, the chemical methods of analysis may require the concentration to be kept as high as possible during the measurements. Since a pure elimination curve is always needed to determine k_{20}, a short intravenous infusion is suggested in cases of doubt.

3. Dost's Rule of Corresponding Fractional Areas

The principle used in the previous section can be extended. It may then be applied at will to continuous and discontinuous modes of administration and to all pharmacokinetic models where neither the model nor the mode of administration has to be capable of mathematical description.

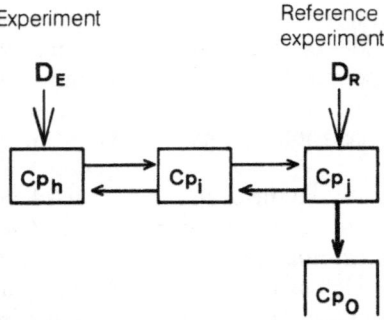

Fig. 31. General pharmacokinetic model to illustrate the Rule of Corresponding Fractional Areas. The ratio of a dose D_E introduced into any given compartment (here Cp_h) can only be described from measurements in the accessible compartment Cp_j (e. g. blood, plasma) when a reference experiment with a dose D_R is carried out in the accessible compartment

Let us first consider Fig. 31: a dose D_E is introduced into compartment h (Cp_h), for example the stomach, by any appropriate route. The behaviour of the dose introduced has to be deduced entirely from measurements in Cp_j, here the blood.

As regards the measurement compartment, the total quantity D_v given at any time can be subdivided into four parts whose ratio one to another is time-dependent. Each of these constituents is, however, a part of the total area under the blood concentration-time curve between $t=0$ and $t=\infty$ which corresponds to the total dose.

a) Fractional Quantities and Fractional Areas

The areas considered here are shown in Fig. 32 for two periods of measurement, together with descriptions of those fractional quantities to which they relate. A preliminary experiment in which a sufficiently large dose D_R is given rapidly into the accessible compartment (Cp_j; blood) is necessary to obtain a reference curve for each experiment.

Occupancy is the quantity present in the blood at any time t when it gives rise to a measurable concentration y. The areas which represent it can be calculated in the manner already described so long as the reference curve has a log-linear form.

Transit is the quantity which has reached the blood and then been irretrievably eliminated during the time t. For a substance excreted solely by the kidneys, the amount would be that found at time t in the urine. It is given by the integral of the blood concentration curve from zero time to time t and thus by the area under the curve up to the time of observation. A

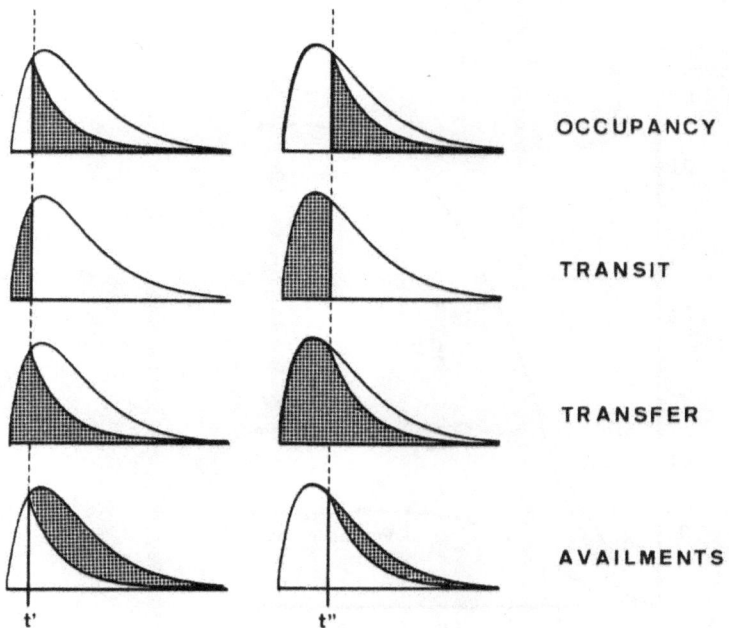

Fig. 32. The corresponding partial areas with a description of their related constituent quantities, shown for two measurement periods, t' and t''

graphical plot of the time course of transit resembles a cumulative excretion curve.

Transfer follows on from the first two terms relating to the steady state as that quantity transported in time t from the compartment of administration Cp_h to the reference compartment Cp_i, i.e. the quantity of substance absorbed. Some of this quantity has been excreted at this time (transit) and some continues to circulate in the blood (occupancy). Its area is therefore the sum of the areas already described and its time course is that of the invasion curve, from which one can recognise whether further compartments between the site of administration and the blood affect invasion.

The invasion curves for oral iron are shown in this manner in Fig. 33. A healthy child absorbs about 22% of the administered dose and this process is virtually complete after 4 h. A child with severe iron deficiency, on the other hand, takes up about 65%. Considerable gastric dilatation with delay in emptying was shown in this child. This may explain the greatly prolonged process of invasion.

Oral iron is known to be used very inefficiently in healthy premature babies. The illustration shows the invasion curve to be not only flatter but also clearly delayed.

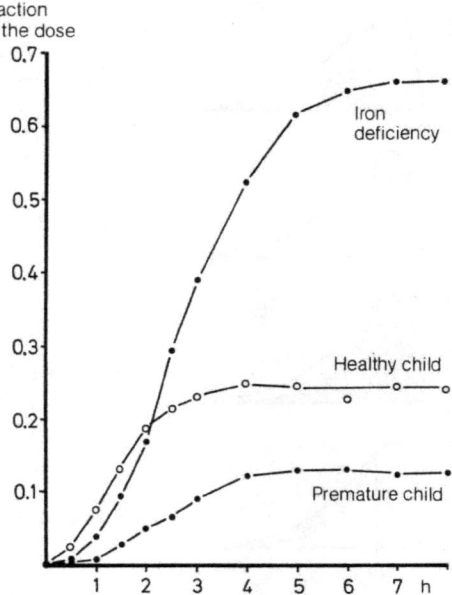

Fig. 33. The absorptions of an iron preparation in three children. Lower curve: premature baby with iron deficiency. Middle curve: healthy girl aged 15 years. Upper curve: dystrophic boy aged 2 years with very severe iron deficiency and marked gastric dilatation. Ordinate: absorbed fraction of the dose. Abscissa: time in hours

Availments are that proportion of the total amount of the substance which has not reached the blood at time t but is *still available for invasion*. They are not therefore the same as the portion of the dose which fails to be taken up over a period because of chemical change at the site of administration or because after being taken by mouth it appears unchanged in the stool. The area representing availments is the difference between the total area S_3 and the area which represents transfer.

b) Conversion of Areas to Quantities of Substance

The equations already expressed can be used to convert areas into amounts of substance even when the mathematical formulation for the basic pharmacokinetic model is not applicable.

The following equation has been applied to a single-compartment model with complete invasion.

$$S = \frac{D}{Cl_{tot}} = \frac{y_0}{k_{20}}. \tag{41}$$

If we designate the time-dependent fractions (1) occupancy (Oc), (2) transit (Ts), (3) transfer (Tf) and (4) availments (Av) collectively as $m_i(t)$ (e.g. milligrams), then the individual quantities are given as the product of each corresponding fractional area $S_i(t)$ and the effective total clearance $\overline{Cl}_{tot}$:

$$m_i(t) = S_i(t) \cdot \overline{Cl}_{tot} \tag{47}$$

This equation is the most general formula for the Rule of Corresponding Areas and it can therefore also be used to determine clearance.

4. General Consideration of Multicompartment Models

The blood concentration-time curve of a drug is often not a straight line on a semilogarithmic plot. This is always so when the curve is the result of the interaction of more than one compartment, as in the Bateman function, where the rate of invasion and the rate of elimination are superimposed.

The same phenomenon will also be observed when distribution in the body is so slow that it cannot be disregarded. A model must then be considered which consists of a 'blood', or, better, a 'central' compartment, and at least one side compartment (Fig. 34).

The combined effect of two compartments gives rise to a biphasic curve: the Bateman function is governed at first by both invasion and elimination but later by the slower of these two processes alone.

When a substance is injected intravenously and is then distributed very slowly outside the blood compartment, the first phase is governed predominantly by elimination and distribution and the later curve by elimination and redistribution. This is frequently referred to as an alpha and a beta phase.

A detailed derivation of the concentration equation from the diagram by means of a series of differential equations is beyond the scope of this book. Simpler and more practical connections must, however, be discussed.

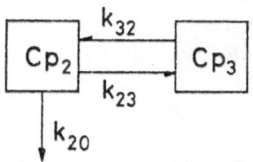

Fig. 34. Two-compartment model with a central compartment (Cp_2) and one side-compartment (Cp_3) which takes up part of the dose reversibly. Intravenous administration would then give rise to a biphasic concentration curve

a) Multi-Exponential Function

A fundamental principle is that the blood concentration-time curve in multicompartment systems may be described mathematically as the sum of as many individual e-functions as there are relevant compartments, i.e. which have a recognisable effect on the curves.

Thus in general:

$$y = \sum_{j=1}^{n} C_j e^{-\gamma_j t}$$

$$= C_1 e^{-\gamma_1 t} + C_2 e^{-\gamma_2 t} \cdots + C_n e^{-\gamma_n t} \qquad (48)$$

where n is the number of compartments which can be recognised and the coefficients C_j and the exponents γ_j are biological constants. They correspond formally to the theoretical initial concentration y_0 and the elimination constant, but they are always compound quantities made up of the constants describing the model (e.g. as noted in the diagram) and are therefore termed hybrid constants. For the model constant k_{ij} itself, the term microconstant has gained acceptance as a way of clarifying differences in terminology.

Thus the general form of the Bateman function, which is determined by $n = 2$ compartments, is:

$$y = \sum_{1}^{2} C_j e^{-\gamma_j t} = C_1 e^{-\gamma_1 t} + C_2 e^{-\gamma_2 t} \qquad (49)$$

with

$$C_1 = \frac{D \cdot k_1}{V(k_2 - k_1)} \quad \text{and} \quad C_2 = -\frac{D \cdot k_1}{V(k_2 - k_1)}$$

We assume for this special case that there is no exchange between the two compartments, but merely an irreversible transfer of the drug from the intramuscular depot into the blood.

Then, and only then, do the following apply:

$$\gamma_1 = k_1 \quad \text{and} \quad \gamma_2 = k_2 \qquad (50)$$

In every case involving several interacting compartments, the exponents (γ_j) will be complex quantities resulting from all the participating transport constants. This makes it difficult to formulate mathematically the relationships which are so clear in the diagram.

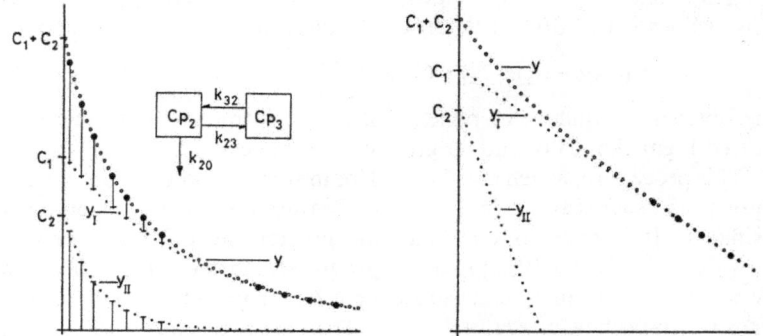

Fig. 35. Biphasic concentration-time curve relating to the model described. From the linear plot (*left*), it is clear that $y = y_I + y_{II}$. In a logarithmic plot (*right*), y_I and y_{II} are straight lines. The curve of the sum of the two does not become a straight line until y_{II} is irrelevant

b) Subdivision into Individual e-Functions

If the n C; γ pairs contained in one blood concentration curve can be determined, then valuable information can be obtained from this which requires no equipment other than that already described.

Figure 35 shows as linear and logarithmic plots the concentration-time curve y for a two-compartment model after intravenous administration:

$$y = C_1 e^{-\gamma_1 t} + C_2 e^{-\gamma_2 t} \tag{51 a}$$

and the two constituent processes:

$$y_1 = C_1 e^{-\gamma_1 t} \quad \text{and} \quad y_{II} = C_2 e^{-\gamma_2 t} \tag{51 b}$$

where $|\gamma_1|$ is smaller than $|\gamma_2|$. The curve approaches a mono-exponential course simply because, as time increases, the process associated with the larger γ vanishes or becomes irrelevant sooner than the slower process, which then controls the situation alone.

The pair of parameters C_1; γ_1 can now be determined in the same way as y_0 and k_2: in the later part of the curve, points are found which can be readily associated with a straight line on a semilogarithmic plot. The intercept of this with the ordinate then gives the value C_1 and its half-time gives the constant γ_1:

$$\gamma_1 = \frac{\ln 2}{t_{50\%1}} \tag{52}$$

If differences are now calculated between the function so obtained and those values which do not lie on this straight line, then, by virtue of

$$y_{II} = (y - C_1 e^{-\gamma_1 t}) = C_2 e^{-\gamma_2 t} \tag{53}$$

one obtains a sequence of points which also form a straight line when plotted logarithmically and so give the parameters C_2; γ_2.

This procedure, which may be used for more than two C; γ-processes, is known as 'successive curve-peeling,' 'feathering' or the 'method of residuals'. It is more operational, the greater the difference between individual values of γ. Because of the progressive formation of differences, the error of determining each subsequent C; γ pair in fact increases with every curve-peeling procedure.

If this procedure is applied to the Bateman function (Fig. 36), the differences y_2 are negative in the ascending part of the curve. They then lie on a curve which tends asymptotically towards the abscissa from *below*. The absolute values of these differences are therefore recorded on the logarithmic scale, taking note of the fact that C_2 must be given a negative sign.

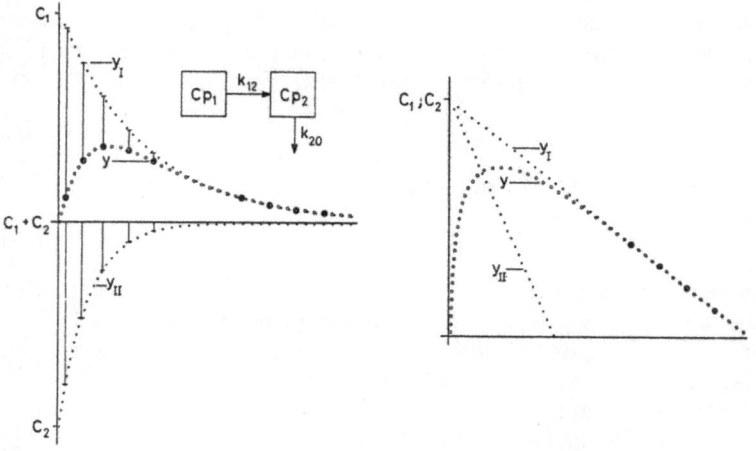

Fig. 36. Biphasic concentration-time course for the Bateman function. On the linear plot (*left*) it is shown as the sum of a positive and a negative exponential function. The initial conditions of y_I and y_{II} have opposing signs but their absolute size is the same. In the logarithmic plot (*right*) the absolute values for $y_{II} = y - y_I$ give a straight line; y only has a linear course when y_{II} can no longer be distinguished from zero

c) Practical Importance of the C; γ-Expression

α) The Half-Time

The method of describing a concentration curve after intravenous injection as the sum of e-functions [Eq. (48)] means that the behaviour of a given drug in the body cannot be characterised by a single half-time. It is however quite usual to give the half-time of the slowest process which is the first C; γ-process to be determined by the curve-peeling procedure:

$$t_{50\%,1} = \frac{\ln 2}{\gamma_1} \tag{54}$$

This is often called the 'biological half-life'. It expresses the fact that, after a certain time, a drug is eliminated from the body (and not only from the blood) at a rate determined exclusively by the slowest C; γ-process. This means that the concentrations in the various compartments are then almost in equilibrium with one another and continue to have a practically constant ratio until elimination is finally complete. This situation is referred to as *pseudo-equilibrium*.

Of course, for clearer characterisation, the half-time of every C; γ-process can be determined. It must, however, be clearly understood that these half-times relate to individual components and not to individual phases or segments of the concentration curve, and that they do not, moreover, describe the behaviour of individual compartments.

β) Areas, Clearance and Elimination Constant

The evaluation of enteric absorption from Eq. (45) may also be applied to multicompartment models. The areas under the total curve are determined as the sum of individual areas which are calculated from each individual C; γ pair according to Eq. (41):

$${}_0^\infty S = \sum \frac{C_j}{\gamma_j} \tag{55}$$

and according to Eq. (41), the total clearance may also be expressed as:

$$Cl_{tot} = \frac{D}{{}_0^\infty S} = \frac{D}{\sum \frac{C_j}{\gamma_j}} \tag{56}$$

This means, however, that the total clearance is even more overestimated when earlier segments of the concentration-time curve are disregarded in the analysis, or where rapid processes are missed because of the timing of blood samples. In such cases the denominator in Eq. (56) is too small by the amount of the disregarded process which equals C/γ.

The actual rate constant of elimination from the blood, the microconstant k_{20}, usually called k_{el} in the British and American literature, can be obtained from

$$k_{20} = \frac{\sum C_j}{\sum \frac{C_j}{\gamma_j}} \tag{57}$$

This rate constant should not, however, be used to calculate a half-time, since it only shows how rapidly the drug would be excreted if there were no side-compartments; k_{20} (or k_{el}), however, expresses the function of the entire system of elimination.

γ) Continuous Intravenous Infusion and the Steady State

If the hybrid constants C_j and γ_j have been determined from the concentration-time curve after intravenous injection of a dose D_{test}, then the curve for continuous intravenous infusion can be obtained for any dosage flow $\dot{D}$ (dose/time)

$$y_{Infusion} = \frac{\dot{D}}{D_{test}} \sum \frac{C_j}{\gamma_j} (1 - e^{-\gamma_j t}) \tag{58}$$

which takes into account the fact that the C_j depends directly on the dose D_{test} used in the basic experiment.

By substituting $t = \infty$ we obtain the steady-state concentration:

$$y^* = \frac{\dot{D}}{D_{test}} \cdot \sum \frac{C_j}{\gamma_j} = \frac{\dot{D}}{Cl_{tot}} \tag{59}$$

We should note here that this concentration depends solely on the dosage flow $\dot{D}$ and the total clearance, and that the rules given in Eq. (46) are independent of the nature of the pharmacokinetic model. For the same total clearance and dosage flow, the infusion curves of various models are distinguished only by their form and not by their limiting states (Fig. 37).

δ) Volumes of Distribution

In multicompartment models, the *total* volume in which the drug can be dissolved is the sum of the compartments. The theoretical initial concentration y_0, which Eq. (48) gives where $t = 0$, that is

$$y_0 = \sum C_j \tag{60}$$

equals zero for extravascular administration. For intravenous administration however, it only relates to that volume in which the dose has been

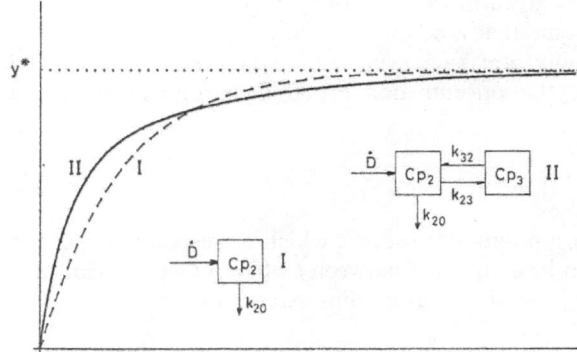

Fig. 37. Continuous intravenous infusion. Comparison of the time course in a model of one (I) and two (II) compartments, assuming the same total clearance. The limiting concentration depends only on the clearance and dosage flow. Hence the classic method of determining clearance by means of chronic infusion can also be used in complicated models. D, dosage flow. Ordinate: concentration (linear scale). Abscissa: time. Both dimensions are in arbitrary units

directly delivered and from which the drug reaches the other compartments by transport, diffusion or by reversible chemical transfer. The size of this *central volume of distribution*

$$V_{central} = \frac{D}{\sum C_j} \tag{61}$$

is always estimated as smaller when blood samples are more frequent, giving a greater number of recognisable C; γ-processes. The smallest central volume of distribution possible is the plasma volume itself (e.g. in situations of very strong binding to plasma protein).

The size of the *total volume of distribution* can also be determined from the C; γ expression. A detailed mathematical analysis of the model, which is often difficult, is not necessary. The procedure is therefore independent of the interrelation of individual compartments, since their sum can be found directly. The concentrations in all compartments in the steady state of continuous intravenous infusion equilibrate completely. This concentration is assumed to be represented by the steady-state concentration y^* in the blood. If the amount of substance M^* producing this concentration is known, then the distribution volume V_{ss} (derived in concept from the steady state) is obtained by definition as

$$V_{ss} = \frac{M^*}{y^*} \tag{62}$$

y^* is given in Eq. (59) and a theoretical experiment provides M^*. If we assume that a continuous infusion (Eq. 58) would be discontinued after equilibrium is achieved, and we put the time of ceasing the infusion as $t=0$, then the concentration from this time onwards would decline according to

$$y = \frac{\dot{D}}{D_{test}} \sum \frac{C_j}{\gamma_j} e^{-\gamma_j t} \tag{63}$$

The amount of substance which corresponded to concentration y^* would then be eliminated between $t=0$ and $t=\infty$. It can thus be determined by the Law of Corresponding Areas [Eq. (46)]:

$$M^* = Cl_{tot} \cdot {}_0^\infty S_{outflow} \tag{64a}$$

$$M^* = Cl_{tot} \frac{\dot{D}}{D_{test}} \sum \frac{C_j}{\gamma_j^2} \tag{64b}$$

This enables V_{ss} to be obtained from the results of a single intravenous injection:

$$V_{ss} = D \cdot \frac{\sum \frac{C_j}{\gamma_j^2}}{\left(\sum \frac{C_j}{\gamma_j}\right)^2} \cdot \tag{65a}$$

$$V_{ss} = V_{cen} \cdot \frac{\sum \frac{C_j}{\gamma_j^2}}{\left(\sum \frac{C_j}{\gamma_j}\right)^2} \cdot \sum C_j \tag{65b}$$

$$V_{ss} = \frac{Cl_{tot}^2}{D} \cdot \sum \frac{C_j}{\gamma_j^2} \tag{65c}$$

$$V_{ss} = Cl_{tot} \frac{\sum \frac{C_j}{\gamma_j^2}}{\sum \frac{C_j}{\gamma_j}} \tag{65d}$$

Experimental factors seldom allow more than two or, for extravascular administration, more than three compartments to be demonstrated unless computers can be used. The description given here may be generally applied, however, and is independent of models, since it is based on the single assumption that elimination is from the central compartment alone.

The work involved in calculation is much simpler in the commonest case involving two compartments than appears at first sight from the equations we have given. Renal function may therefore be determined quite practically by means of inulin, phenol red or chromium-EDTA clearances, which relate to a two-compartment model, instead of by continuous infusion [Eq. (58)], by single intravenous or even single intramuscular injection [Eq. (40)].

VI. Pharmacokinetics and Treatment

We have concentrated up to now on descriptive and analytical aspects of pharmacokinetics and have seen how the behaviour of individual drugs in the human body can be characterised by quantitative expressions, independently of their pharmacological and toxicological properties. We have also seen how the pharmacokinetic indices for suitable test substances can describe the function of organs and organ systems. *Pharmacokinetics is thus a valuable clinical tool for physiological and pathological research and forms the basis of many routine procedures for organ function tests.*

This section is concerned with practical questions related to the use of drugs.

The effectiveness of a drug depends on its concentration at the active site on the receptor. This applies not only to those receptors whose pharmacological activities evoke the desired therapeutic effect but also to those which express an alteration of their state by toxic manifestations. The same receptors may be involved in both cases. In the drugs used in practice, however, there is a quantitative difference between the concentration needed for therapeutic activity and the maximal concentration tolerable on account of toxicity. The ratio of these two concentrations is a measure of the therapeutic range of a drug.

The minimal effective concentration of most antimicrobial agents is precisely known. For other drugs, one at least knows at what blood concentration a pharmacological effect begins to occur.

The amount of a substance which must be given in order to achieve the desired concentration may be readily calculated from the volume of distribution and the concentration required. If the therapeutic range of the substance is known, the maximum tolerable dose can also be obtained. It is not generally sufficient merely to achieve the necessary concentration in the blood and at the receptor sites. This concentration must also be maintained for an adequate period, which is only possible by achieving steady-state conditions, as discussed in Section IV. In practice, however, a single dose is generally given which is sufficient to produce blood concentrations that exceed the therapeutic minimum by a tolerable amount, so achieving an adequate concentration for a longer period. This principle is used in long-acting and ultra-long-acting preparations, e.g. some sulphonamides, tetracyclines and barbiturates, where the delay is due to very slow excretion, the half-life being of the order of days.

Another approach is to use depot preparations where invasion is greatly delayed when an appropriate galenic preparation is chosen. For crystalline suspensions such as benzathine penicillin and some corticosteroids, the solubility of the drug in tissue water at the site of administration is the rate-determining step. Diffusion within the solvent controls the rate for oily preparations. Some oral preparations are available whose active constituents are sequestered in layers of differing solubility, or are released in a delayed fashion by an ion exchanger, so that invasion is also delayed (slow-release preparations).

1. Repeated Administration of a Drug

The opportunities for treatment with long-acting and depot preparations are limited, however, and repeated doses must usually be given. Obviously, the larger each single dose, the longer the necessary minimal concentration is exceeded. The size of each individual dose may well be limited by toxicity, however.

The values for the minimal effective concentration, the possible toxic concentration and the half-time of elimination determine the limits of rational dosage since, with the exception of depot preparations, the invasion of most drugs is so rapid that it may in practice be disregarded for these purposes. In the next section it will therefore be assumed that conditions of intravenous administration pertain.

a) Duration of Accumulation

ne exponential law of elimination states that the concentration of a substance delivered into the blood will eventually fall below a predetermined minimal concentration after a calculable time, but that it will only reach zero after infinite time.

Table 3 shows how much of a drug remains in the body at various times after intravenous administration when the half-time of elimination is chosen as the time unit. The equation already given for elimination

$$y = y_0 e^{-k_2 t} \tag{5}$$

thus becomes

$$y = y_0 e^{-\varepsilon \ln 2} = y_0 2^{-\varepsilon} \qquad \varepsilon = \frac{t}{t_{50\%}} \tag{66}$$

Such a table is very useful for a number of dosage problems. It is easily extended by successive multiplication: for increments of ε of 0.01, each number is the product of $0.9931 = 2^{-0.01}$ and the figure which immediately precedes it. For increments of 0.1, the factor is 0.9330, and for 1.0, it is 0.5. Intermediate values which are not in Table 3, e.g. 4.31, are given by:

$$2^{-4.31} = 2^{-4} \cdot 2^{-0.3} \cdot 2^{-0.01} = 0.0625 \cdot 0.8123 \cdot 0.9931 = 0.0504$$

Table 3 applies to all substances that are excreted exponentially, and shows clearly that it depends purely on the dose and the time based on the half-time of elimination, whether the residual amount to which the new dose is always added in intermittent dosing is therapeutically effective or toxic.

As an example to clarify the use of the table, let us assume that phenylbutazone, which has a half-time of elimination of about 69 h, is to be given in equal doses D every 8 h, as is the usual clinical practice. The dose interval is thus

$$\tau = \varepsilon \cdot t_{50\%} = 8 \text{ h}$$
$$\varepsilon = \frac{8}{69} = 0.13$$

The table shows that a residue from the first dose of $D \cdot 0.9138$ is still present in the body immediately before the second dose. Since the second dose is added to this, the peak concentration which follows it is determined by the amount

$$D \cdot 0.9138 + D = D \cdot 1.9138$$

Table 3. Table of values for the function $y = 2^{-\varepsilon}$. ε is a time unit based on the half-time $t_{50\%}$ of a drug

ε	$2^{-\varepsilon}$	ε	$2^{-\varepsilon}$	ε	$2^{-\varepsilon}$
0.00	1.0000	0.00	1.0000	0.00	1.00000
0.01	0.9931	0.10	0.9330	1.00	0.50000
0.02	0.9862	0.20	0.8706	2.00	0.25000
0.03	0.9794	0.30	0.8123	3.00	0.12500
0.04	0.9727	0.40	0.7579	4.00	0.06250
0.05	0.9659	0.50	0.7071	5.00	0.03125
0.06	0.9593	0.60	0.6598	6.00	0.01563
0.07	0.9526	0.70	0.6156	7.00	0.00781
0.08	0.9461	0.80	0.5743	8.00	0.00391
0.09	0.9395	0.90	0.5359	9.00	0.00195
0.10	0.9330	1.00	0.5000	10.00	0.00098

Immediately after the third dose, i.e. $2\varepsilon t_{50\%}$ after the first dose, its residue is $D \cdot 0.8351$, and that from the second dose is $D \cdot 0.9138$, and to these remainders the third dose must be added. The total amount present in the body is then

$$D \cdot 0.8351 + D \cdot 0.9138 + D = D \cdot 2.7489$$

This calculation can be continued for each subsequent dose. Thus it is the quantity still remaining from the *first* dose only that must be determined for each repetition of the dose and added as the new component. We now know that the residual accumulation and hence also the peak concentration only increase visibly so long as sufficient of the first dose is still present in the body.

Bearing in mind that after four half-times of elimination, 93.75% of a single dose will have been excreted, it is clear that, even after repeated dosage, no marked increase in the cumulative residue is to be expected after this time. This means for phenylbutazone that, after $4 \times 69 = 276$ h ($= 11.5$ days), the cumulative residue and maximal concentration will have reached 93.75% of that value which can be achieved by continuous therapy. How long such an increase with repeated administration is clinically relevant depends purely on the half-time of elimination.

b) Degree of Accumulation

The degree of accumulation is a function of the number of doses per half-time of elimination and therefore of the relative dose-interval

$$\varepsilon = \frac{\tau}{t_{50\%}}; \quad (\tau = \text{dose-interval}) \tag{67}$$

When a dose D is given an infinite number of times at intervals of $\tau = \varepsilon \cdot t_{50\%}$, the amount of drug present in the body immediately after a dose is

$$M_{max} = D \frac{1}{1 - e^{-k_2 \tau}} = D \frac{1}{1 - 2^{-\varepsilon}} \tag{68}$$

The cumulative residue immediately before this and every subsequent dose is smaller by the exact value of D:

$$M_{min} = M_{max} - D = D \left(\frac{1}{1 - 2^{-\varepsilon}} - 1 \right) \tag{69}$$

For phenylbutazone, whose half-time is 69 h, $\varepsilon = 0.13$ when doses are given every 8 h. By substituting the appropriate values from Table 3,

$$M_{max} = D \cdot \frac{1}{1 - 0.9138} = D \cdot 11.61$$

and so

$$M_{max} = D \cdot (11.61 - 1) = D \cdot 10.61$$

This means that repeated doses of phenylbutazone at 8-hourly intervals lead finally to a limiting maximal value which is 11.6 times higher than the highest value after a single dose, and that the minimal value remaining at the end of a dose interval is still 10.6 times as high. The physician must decide whether this is what he wants.

M_{min}, on the other hand, is the exact amount which needs to be added to the initial dose at constant dosage in order to establish the effect of accumulation present at the outset. M_{min} is therefore analogous to the priming dose *D from Section IV.

A further useful relationship can be derived from Eqs. (68) and (69):

$$\frac{M_{max}}{M_{min}} = \frac{1}{e^{-k_2 \tau}} = \frac{1}{2^{-\varepsilon}} \tag{70}$$

Table 3 now enables us to test whether the fluctuations in the steady state at a planned relative dose interval ε still lie safely within the therapeutic range of the drug [Eq. (67)].

Although strictly speaking the conditions of Eqs. (68) and (69) only apply to the intravenous route, they nevertheless give a useful concept for

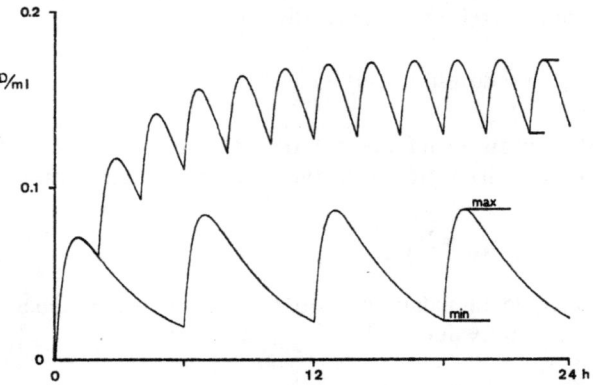

Fig. 38. The concentration-time curve for sparteine when 0.1 dose units/volume of distribution are given repeatedly. The dose intervals are 2 h (upper curve) and 6 h (lower curve). After 8 h, changes in the max/min ratio are very small. Ordinate: concentration in dose units/volume of distribution. Abscissa: time in hours

non-intravenous administration, since k_1 for most substances is considerably greater than k_2.

The practical importance of accumulation is also illustrated by an example of oral administration.

Figure 38 shows the effect of the dose interval on the height of the blood concentrations of sparteine. The half-time of invasion is 0.2 h and that of elimination, 1.9 h. With 4 daily doses at 6-h intervals, there is virtually no accumulation after the first dose and the max/min ratio is 3.9, which is greater than the therapeutic range of the drug. When given every 2 h, max/min = 1.3, which would be tolerable; 2-hourly dosage over a long period is not, however, a practical proposition for the patient.

Studying the effect of repetitive dosage on the blood concentration in a system with two or more compartments is laborious and only really possible with the aid of automatic calculators or even analogue computers, as in the above case. This procedure will be discussed later.

In multicompartment systems, each C; γ-process is treated in such a way that it represents the concentration-time curve of a drug on its own. The results of all the C; γ-processes are summated for each time at which an estimate of accumulation is required. It should not, however, be forgotten that processes with a negative C occur with extravascular administration which, when considered in isolation, can accumulate negatively. Although at first sight this seems complicated, it solves the problem of the exact calculation of accumulation in the bloodstream.

VII. Pharmacokinetics of Gastrointestinal Absorption*

Some new factors have to be taken into account when considering the pharmacokinetics of blood concentration-time curves of substances absorbed through the gastrointestinal tract. These are: 1) the amount of substance which can be absorbed varies with gastrointestinal filling and emptying; 2) invasion into the circulation often does not obey the laws of simple concentration gradients; 3) the interposition of organs of active metabolism such as the liver or intestinal mucosa can lead to a partial or complete change in the substance absorbed; 4) counter-regulatory influences may affect substances absorbed in the gastrointestinal tract, particularly foodstuffs.

All of these processes of concentration may in principle be incorporated into suitably formulated models. This results in a multiple but discontinuous system of formulae of which a simple example is discussed in the next section. Such detailed analysis of the curves, which is only accurate when larger computers are used, is rarely necessary in practice. We must nevertheless keep in mind the numerous variables in enteric absorption in order to avoid applying ready-made computer programmes to substances whose properties of absorption are imperfectly understood.

It is advisable, therefore, to begin the study of gastrointestinal absorption without resorting to preconceived models. Lengthy calculations can be avoided by reconstructing the invasion curve (Kübler, 1970). We will therefore consider this procedure here. The more important formulae and those derivations of them which are unavoidable are summarised in an appendix to this chapter.

1. Gastrointestinal Absorption and the Bateman Function

The similarity between the concentration-time curve for gastrointestinal absorption and that for the Bateman function can be very misleading. The

---

* By W. Kübler, Giessen. Dedicated to Prof. Dr. h. c. Franz Klose, Kiel, on the occasion of his 85th birthday, 21st July, 1972.

two only coincide satisfactorily when the invasion constants and passage time for the segment of intestine where absorption occurs are large enough; their product must be at least 3.5 in order that a minimum of 97% of the substance delivered is absorbed. The initial part of the curve is determined by that time at which all the substance being absorbed has reached the intestinal segment where absorption occurs. It therefore depends largely on the kinetics of gastric emptying.

A computer programme set up by Krüger-Thiemer and Eriksen (1966) exploits the similarity between the gastrointestinal absorption curves and the Bateman function; it determines the invasion constants of the curves but ignores the flattened-off initial portion (Fig. 39, *hatched area*). The equations so far derived show that this procedure gives reliable results only when the invasion constant and passage time permit almost complete absorption, which is unfortunately seldom the case.

The example chosen for Figs. 39, 41 and 43 should make this clear: the Bateman function only satisfactorily approximates to the model curve when t_2 is 5 h or more (*dotted line*). It only coincides with the nearby concentration-time curve over the short segment between t_1 and t_2, and only one measurement has been made in this region.

Short gastric emptying times such as are brought about by heavy fluid loads in the fasting state make it easier to evaluate the absorption curves by this programme. In every case one must test whether the amount of substance absorbed increases proportionally with increasing dose; if this

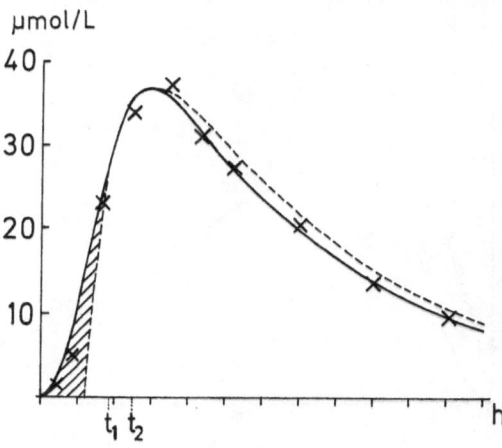

Fig. 39. Plasma sulphonamide concentrations following 4 g sulphathiourea. X, values measured; ———, curve calculated from Eq. (83 a–d) (cf. Figs. 43, 45 and 49); $k_2 = 0.177$, $k_1 = 1.175$, $t_1 = 1.85$, $t_2 = 2.5$; ‐ ‐ ‐ ‐ ‐ ‐ ‐ ‐, Bateman function with the same constants of elimination and invasion

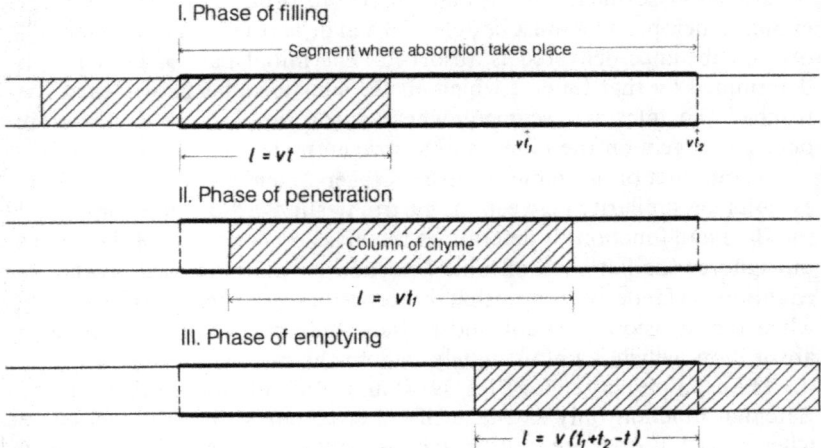

Fig. 40. Phases of absorption which result from the position of the substance in relation to the segment of intestine where absorption occurs

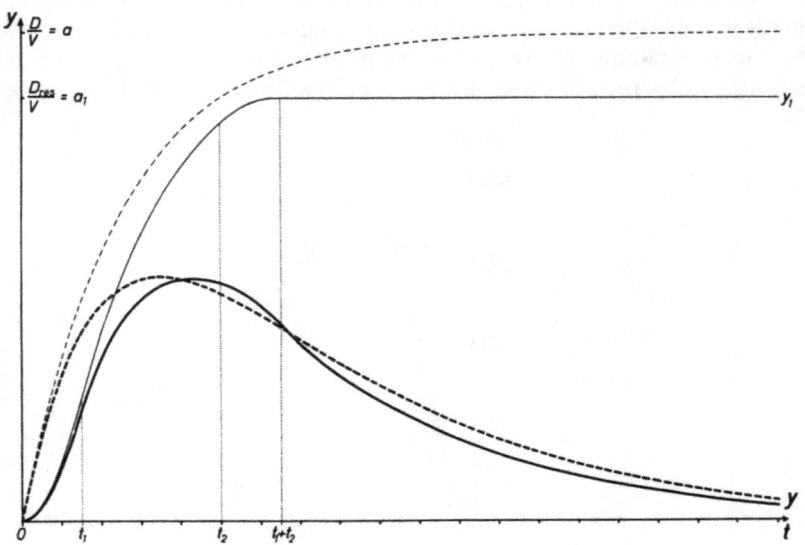

Fig. 41. Invasion- and concentration-time curves of dose-proportional gastrointestinal absorption (———) in comparison with the Bateman function (– – – – – – –). y, concentration curves; y_1, invasion curves; abscissa units: hours. For both curves, $k_1 = 0.4\ h^{-1}$; $k_2 = 0.2\ h^{-1}$

does not occur, invasion constants no longer apply because a saturation function has replaced the Bateman function and this can be better calculated with the aid of the Michaelis-Menten equation. A simple model clarifies the nature of the distortion of the Bateman function by the filling and emptying of the section of bowel in which absorption occurs (Fig. 40). The first assumption is that the substance is distributed uniformly in a cylindrical column of chyme which passes at a uniform rate (v) through a hollow cylinder in which absorption occurs. The cylinder of chyme is assumed (for the moment) as being of constant length. Two time constants are involved, namely the *filling time* (t_1), which is the time needed by the cylinder of chyme to enter the absorbing area of intestine completely (thereby giving a cylinder length $l = v \cdot t_1$), and the *passage time* (t_2) after which the chyme cylinder moves away from the intestinal segment where absorption occurs.

Three phases of absorption can therefore be recognised which precede the phase of pure decline in the blood concentration-time curve for absorption, namely

I. The *phase of filling* ($0 \leq t \leq t_1$). The quantity of absorbable substrate increases uniformly until at t_1 the entire column of chyme lies in the intestinal segment where absorption occurs.

II. The *phase of penetration* ($t_1 \leq t \leq t_2$). Between t_1 and t_2 absorption can occur from the entire cylinder of chyme.

III. The *phase of emptying* ($t_2 \leq t \leq t_1 + t_2$). After t_2 the column of chyme moves away from the absorbing segment of intestinal mucosa.

IV. The *phase of decline* ($t \geq t_1 + t_2$). Absorption has ended; the subsequent course of the invasion- and concentration-time curves is determined by the reactions of the absorbed substrate.

The invasion and concentration-time curves for various conditions of absorption can be derived from this model. The simplest case of absorption which is proportional to the dose is formulated in the appendix [Eqs. (82 a–d) and (83 a–d)] and contrasted in Figs. 39 and 41 with a Bateman function with corresponding characteristics. This comparison shows that the *phase of filling* affects the entire course of the curve. During the *phase of penetration* from t_1 to t_2, the Bateman function applies, although changed in form by another combination of constants. In the *phase of emptying*, the invasion and concentration curves level off more than the Bateman function and absorption is then likely to be practically at an end. It is particularly important to note that during the *phase of decline* for the simple process of absorption, a strictly exponentially declining concentration curve must emerge, in contrast to the Bateman function which approximates asymptotically to such a time course. Phase IV of the equation for invasion shows the final state of absorption.

Quantitatively:

$$D_{abs} = D(1 - e^{-k_1 t_2}) \tag{71}$$

This means that where the amount of substance absorbed (D_{abs}) is proportional to the dose (D), D_{abs} depends only on the invasion constant (k_1) and the passage time (t_2) for the intestinal segment where absorption occurs. The simplified assumptions of a uniform rate of penetration by food (v), a constant length, and a concentration in the intestinal contents which is altered only by the process of absorption are *not*, therefore, requirements for the correctness of the model. This is not so surprising, since the surface of the column and the concentration in it, which are the most important factors in absorption, will be affected in opposite senses by variations in the volume of the cylinder. Since both of the above factors affect the rate of absorption linearly, increasing or decreasing the amount of fluid in the column does not affect absorption so long as the latter is proportionally related to the dose.

2. Reconstruction of the Invasion Curves

The previous chapters have shown in detail that a blood concentration-time curve is the result of two opposing processes, invasion and elimination. The superimposition of elimination makes it extremely difficult to assess or compare the underlying processes of absorption when the rate constants of elimination are different. It is certainly an advantage, therefore, to adjust the superimposed processes of elimination by use of a calculator or computer and thus to show the invasion curve in isolation. If the elimination constant (k_2) is known (and does not vary) then the following statement can be applied to any given blood concentration-time curve: the quantity of substance eliminated [$y_{el}(t)$] (expressed as a concentration in the volume of distribution) up to the time of measurement t must be added to any measured value [$y(t)$], as follows:

$$y_1(t) = y(t) + y_{el}(t) \tag{72}$$

As with the Rule of Corresponding Areas, $y_{el}(t)$ is determined by the elimination constant (k_2) and the area under the blood concentration-time curve (i.e. from an integral $\int_0^t y \, dt$). Thus, from Eq. (72),

$$y_1(t) = y(t) + k_2 \int_0^t y \, dt \tag{73}$$

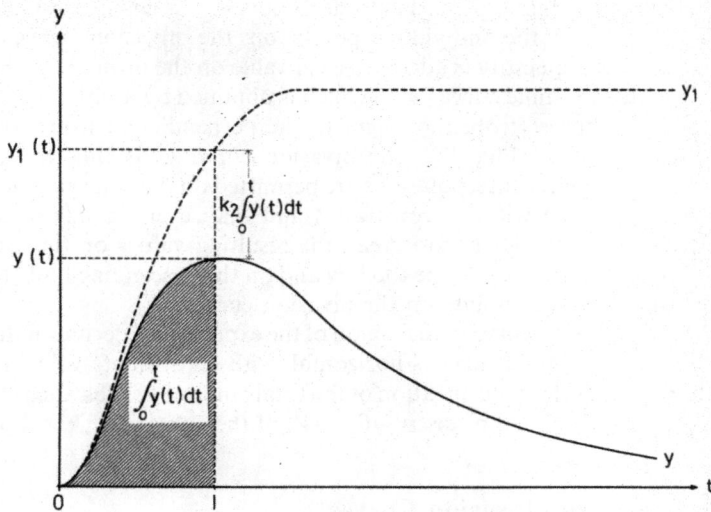

Fig. 42. Reconstruction of the invasion curve (y_1) from a concentration-time curve (y) according to Eq. (73)

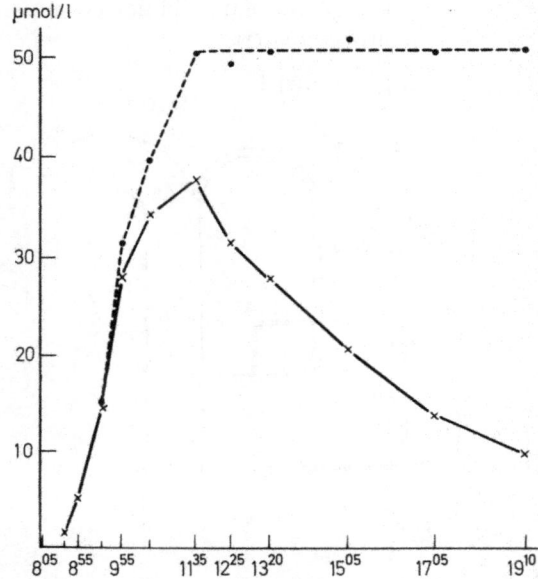

Fig. 43. Serum concentration and invasion curve after 4 g sulphathiourea (*cf.* Fig. 39)

This statement is proved in the appendix to this chapter. Equation (73) indicates how the individual points on the invasion curve can be calculated: a quantity is added to each value on the ordinate of the blood concentration-time curve $[y(t)]$ which is obtained by multiplying the area under the curve [from the origin to the perpendicular from $y(t)$ to the abscissa] by k_2 (Fig. 42). The invasion curve y_1 is thus made up of individual points. Interpolations are permitted on the concentration curve (where possible without constraint) and may even be advisable since, where the intervals are too great, the resulting values on the ascending portion of the curve may be too low and on the descending limb, too high for the associated points on the invasion curve.

The invasion curve in the region of the exponential decline in the blood concentration-time curve is horizontal, with an ordinate value a_1 which characterises the concentration of the total amount of substance absorbed (D_{abs}) in the volume of distribution (V) of the substance (Fig. 43).

3. Use of the Invasion Curves

Quantitative evidence about the amount of substance $[D_{abs}(t)]$ which passes into the systemic circulation at any particular instant (t) is given by the product of the volume of distribution (V) and the value of the ordinate $[y_1(t)]$ on the invasion curve

$$D_{abs}(t) = y_1(t) \, V \tag{74}$$

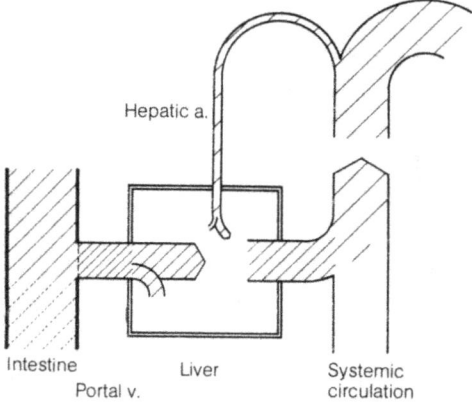

Fig. 44. Diagram to show the retention of substrate by the liver from the portal blood and systemic circulation

Evidence of the amount of substance absorbed from the intestine or peritoneal cavity is only given by Eq. (74), however, when the fraction of the absorbed substrate to be retained by the liver from the portal blood (first-pass effect) is known (Fig. 44). For this purpose, the distribution spaces, or else the urinary excretion of the substance after both forms of administration, can be compared. Further details are given by calculations from Eq. (71).

Qualitative evidence, especially the parameters governing intestinal absorption, can be calculated directly from the invasion curve; these calculations are not affected by the retention of substance by the liver so long as it is in proportion to the dose, which is usually the case. The invasion constant (k_{12}) is most simply obtained by calculation from the graph. The invasion curves for gastrointestinal absorption can, moreover, be converted by calculating the difference between the values on the ascending limb of the curve and the final horizontal value ($a - y_1$), plotted semilogarithmically.

From these quantities, we obtain

$$a - y_1 = C^* \cdot e^{-k_1 t} \qquad (75)$$

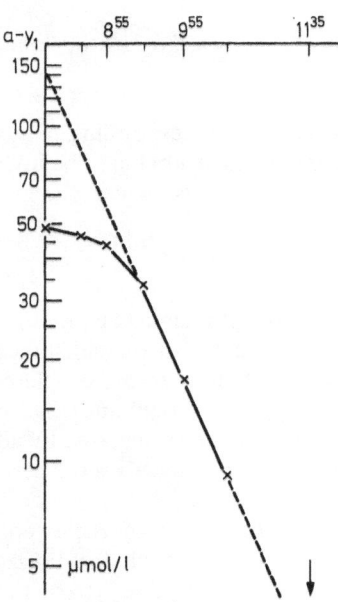

Fig. 45. Invasion curve after 4 g sulphathiourea, plotted on a log-linear scale as the differences from the final concentration (a). *Cf.* Fig. 43

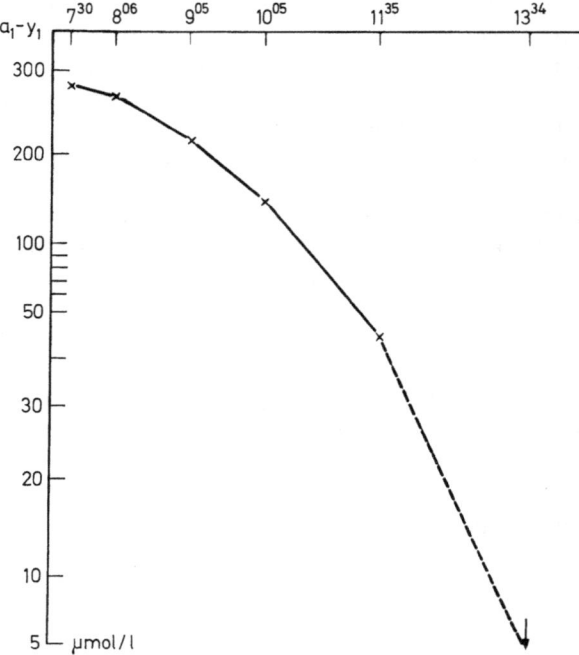

Fig. 46. Invasion after 3 g ascorbic acid (48% absorption)

where C^* (corresponding to y_0) is the intercept with the ordinate on the extended invasion line. The invasion constant (k_{10}) can then be calculated from Eq. (7) just as can the rate constant of elimination (k_{20}):

$$k_{12} = \frac{\ln(a - y_1(t_1)) - \ln(a - y_1(t_2))}{t_2 - t_1} \tag{76}$$

Absorption must be practically complete for this statement to apply. If more than 8% of the substance administered is not absorbed, then the curve obtained from the differences $(a - y_1)$ and plotted semilogarithmically is not a straight line (Fig. 46). When enough measurements have been made, a may be calculated by adding a constant value to all points on the curve in order to obtain the best approximation to a straight line on a log-linear plot.

In the region of the exponentially declining terminal part of the absorption curve (which is horizontal in the invasion curve), the position of each calculated value $y_1(t)$ on the terminal horizontal without distortion in

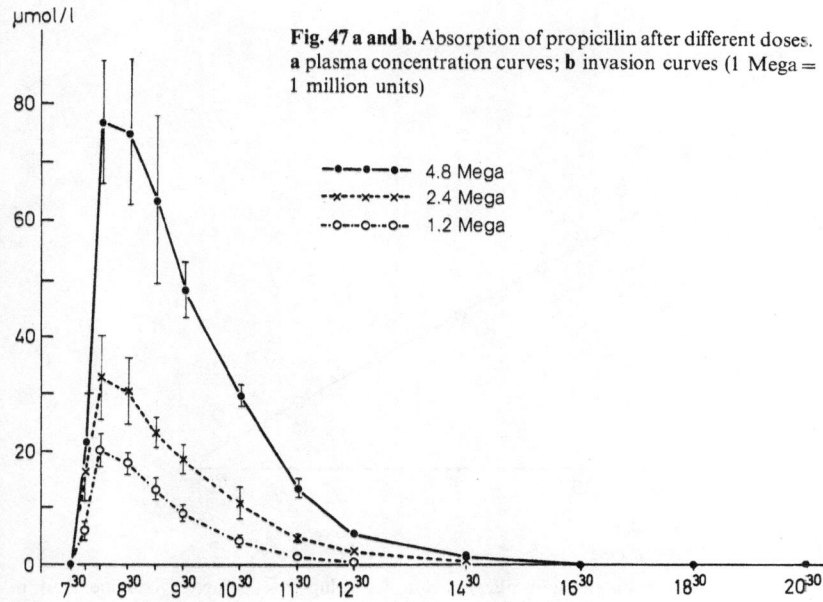
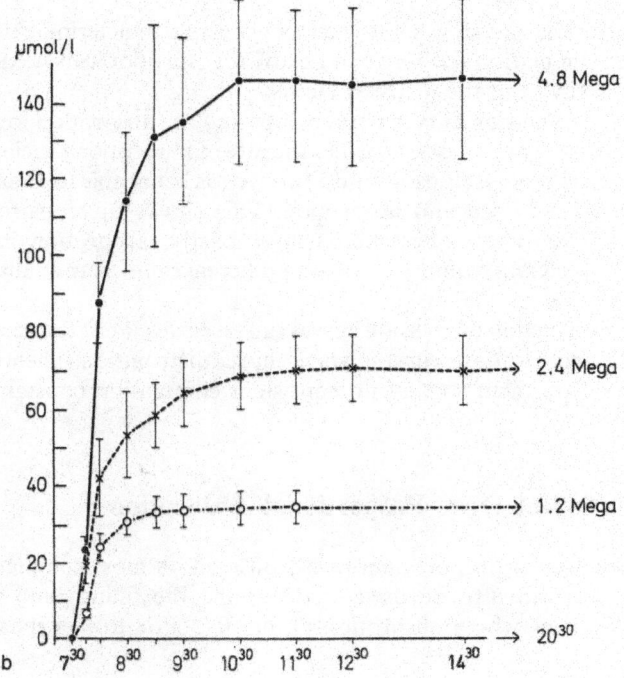

Fig. 47 a and b. Absorption of propicillin after different doses. **a** plasma concentration curves; **b** invasion curves (1 Mega = 1 million units)

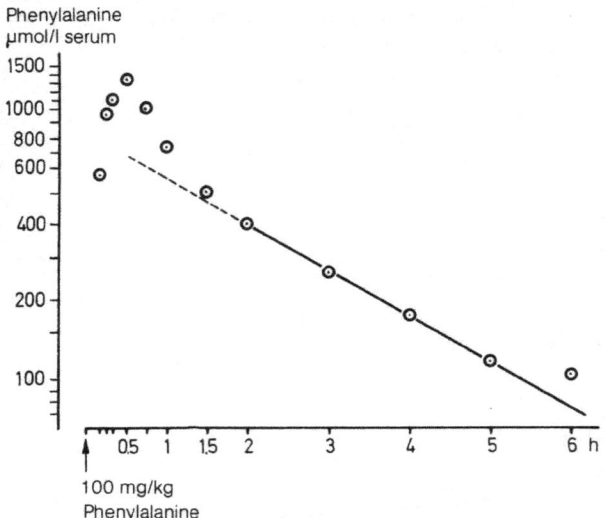

Fig. 48. Biphasic distribution phenomenon following an oral phenylalanine load of 100 mg/kg

a semilogarithmic plot shows how well we were able to determine the rate constant of elimination (*cf.* Fig. 43). Lastly, reabsorption can be quantitated very easily from the invasion curve.

By plotting invasion curves when comparing the absorption found at different dosage, we can assess whether the rate of absorption is delayed in any phase of the process (Figs. 47 and 54) as well as being able to quantitate the ratio between dose and absorption. This shows up impaired absorption due to rapid intestinal passage. Lastly, absorption can be compared in different volunteers despite differences in their elimination constants.

The reconstruction of invasion curves can be *misleading* if they are used on blood concentration curves which have distribution phenomena superimposed on them so that no consistent elimination constants are found (Fig. 48).

4. Calculation of Dose-Proportional Absorption

When absorption is proportional to the dose and almost complete, the invasion curve can also be used to determine the filling time of the intestinal segment where absorption occurs (t_1). For this purpose, the

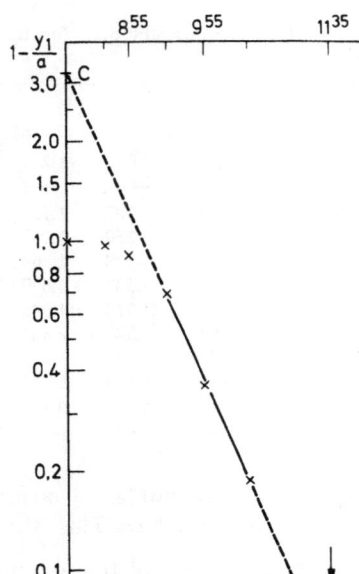

Fig. 49. Invasion curve following 4 g sulphathiourea, according to $1 - (y_1 : a)$, plotted semilogarithmically. C can be used to calculate t_1 (cf. Fig. 45)

invasion curve is adjusted by putting the final horizontal portion $(a_1) = 1$ and expressing the individual points $[y_1(t)]$ as fractions of the final value $\frac{y_1}{a}$; a can of course be calculated from $ln(a_1 - y_1)$, as described earlier. The difference from 1 is plotted semilogarithmically (Fig. 49) just as for the invasion curve:

$$1 - \frac{y_1}{a} = C \cdot e^{-k_1 t} \quad \text{for} \quad t_1 \leqq t \leqq t_2 \tag{77}$$

C is determined by two constants, k_1 and t_1 (see Sect. 7 of this chapter for derivation):

$$C = \frac{e^{k_1 t_1} - 1}{k_1 t_1} \tag{78}$$

Since k_1, and C can be calculated, t_1 can be found with their aid.

---

[1] C cannot be determined with sufficient accuracy from a graph, so the intercepts on the ordinate are intentionally calculated from the invasion constants and a point on the invasion curve where on a semilogarithmic plot it forms a straight line:

$$C = \left(1 - \frac{y_1(t)}{a}\right) e^{+k_1 t} \quad \text{for} \quad t_1 \leqq t \leqq t_2 \tag{77a}$$

Table 4. Extract from a table of the function $C = \dfrac{e^{k_1 t_1} - 1}{k_1 t_1}$ for determining t_1 when k_1 and C are known

t_1	k_1						
	0.8	1.0	1.2	1.4	1.6	1.8	2.0
0.2	1.084	1.107	1.130	1.154	1.179	1.204	1.230
0.4	1.179	1.230	1.283	1.340	1.401	1.464	1.532
0.6	1.283	1.370	1.464	1.567	1.679	1.801	1.933
0.8	1.401	1.532	1.679	1.844	2.029	2.237	2.471
1.0	1.532	1.718	1.933	2.182	2.471	2.805	3.195
1.5	1.933	2.321	2.805	3.412	4.176	5.141	6.362
2.0	2.471	3.195	4.176	5.516	7.353	9.888	13.400
2.5	3.195	4.473	6.362	9.176	13.400	19.782	29.483
3.0	4.176	6.361	9.888	15.640	25.106	40.816	67.072

Equation (78) cannot be solved for t_1 and must therefore be determined by an iterative procedure. This is not difficult to do with a programmable calculator. A table of the function $C = \dfrac{e^{k_1 t_1} - 1}{k_1 t_1}$ (Table 4) facilitates the approximation to the unknown value for t_1.

Example: From Fig. 49, $k_1 \simeq 1.175$ and $C \simeq 3.572$. For $k_1 = 1.2$ and $C = 2.805$, Table 4 gives a value of 1.5 h for t_1.

For $k_1 = 1.175$ and $t_1 = 1.5$, $C \simeq 2.739$, and for $t_1 = 2.0$, $C \simeq 4.036$. Linear interpolation gives $C \simeq 3.572$ for $t_1 = 1.82$; a further interpolation gives $t_1 \simeq 1.85$ as the best approximation. Figure 39 shows that, using these parameters, the curves approximate satisfactorily to the points measured.

5. Variants of the Invasion Process in Gastrointestinal Absorption

a) Variants in the Site of Absorption

In simultaneous loads with substances of known absorption characteristics, variants in the site of absorption may be shown by differences in the time parameter t_1. When the substance is absorbed through the gastric mucosa, the value for t_1 is shorter than for substances whose absorption is predominantly duodenal. A prolonged t_1 needs more careful study; besides the fact that absorption may not begin until the deeper segments of intestine are reached, the onset of enzymatic reactions or the solution of the substance may be delayed, giving rise to this effect.

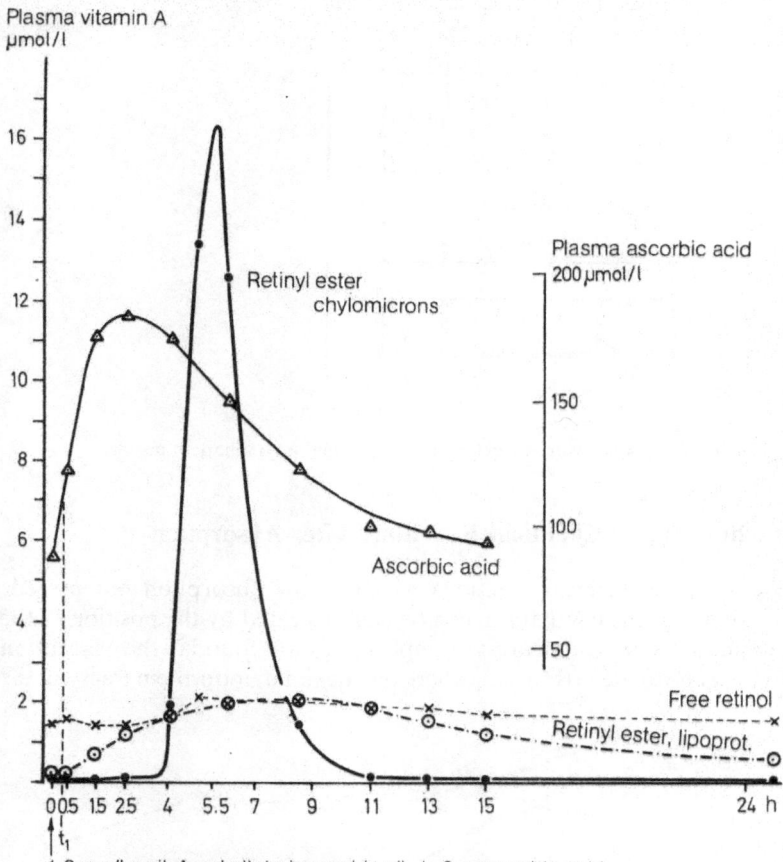

Fig. 50. Retinyl ester in the plasma following a dose of 1.8 mg/kg vitamin A palmitate in an oily solution. Simultaneous dosing of 3 g ascorbic acid to determine t_1

b) Delay in Invasion Due to Lymphatic Transport of Lipid-Soluble Substances

Similar prolongations of the t_1 values are caused by delay in invasion due to lymphatic transport of lipid-soluble substances (Fig. 50). After giving vitamin A palmitate in oil, for example, we were not able to observe the inflow of the predominant chylomicron fraction until after a delay of several hours (Fig. 51). The time interval (t_L) can be calculated and compared with t_1 for ascorbic acid when given simultaneously.

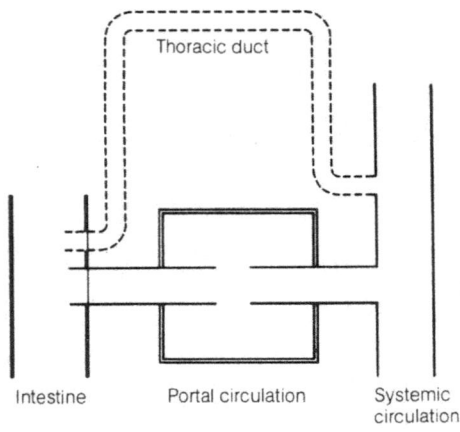

Fig. 51. Flow chart showing the delay in invasion due to lymphatic transport

c) Physical and Chemical Reactions After Absorption

Physical and chemical reactions which follow absorption but precede invasion into the circulation, can be demonstrated by the position of the maximum value. The clearest example of this was found in the absorption curves of β-carotene (Fig. 52), where the maximal lipoprotein fraction, the

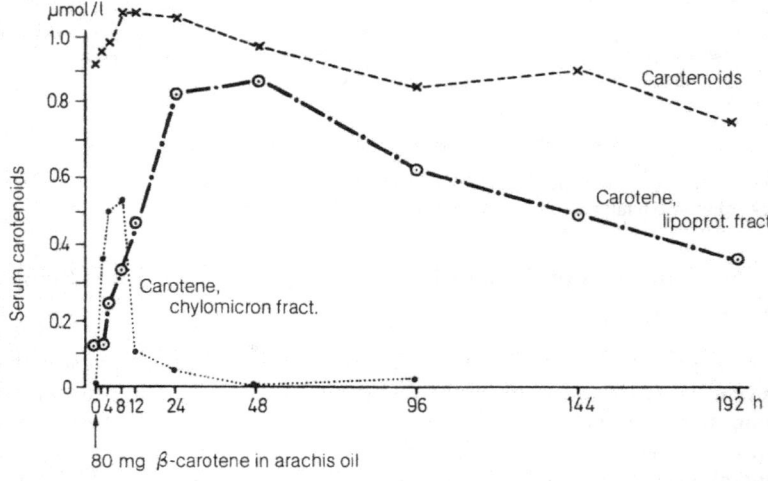

Fig. 52. Plasma carotene concentration after 80 mg β-carotene in arachis oil in adults

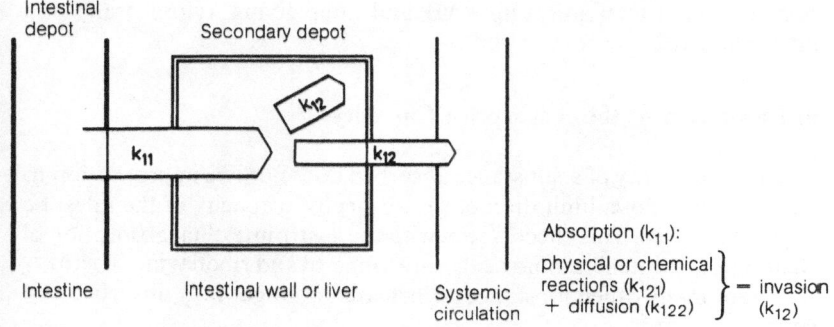

Fig. 53. Flow chart of a 'secondary depot' through a reaction between the intestinal absorption and the invasion of the systemic circulation

principal carrier of the absorbed pro-vitamin, appeared after 24–48 h, which is long after absorption must have been complete, since carotene is absorbed exclusively in the small intestine. The deposition of the pro-vitamin in lipoproteins is the delaying factor here. Circulatory invasion is determined no longer by the rate constant of absorption (k_{11}) but more likely by deposition (k_{121}) on the protein bodies (Fig. 53). Despite incomplete absorption, the similarity with the Bateman function is now much greater [Eq. (40)].

The interposition of such conversion reactions acts as a depot which takes up the absorbed substance at first and then, in accordance with a kinetic constant (k_{12}), returns it to the circulation (the secondary depot phenomenon; formula given in Sect. 7 of this chapter).

d) Excretion and Reabsorption of Substances in the Intestine

The computation may be interfered with considerably by excretion and reabsorption of substances in the intestine, since this is superimposed on the elimination curve. Dost and Repges (1968) observed this after the intravenous administration of bromsulphalein (see Fig. 4) and obtained a good approximation of the curve using a three-compartment model. Such a calculation would be considerably more difficult if such excretion processes were to be superimposed on the absorption curve of an oral substance, since a rate constant of elimination could not then be determined directly; a number of excretion and absorption cycles may be superimposed on the descending limb to such an extent that a considerably lower elimination constant is sometimes substituted. Similar effects have been observed after injecting PAH and after giving xylose orally and intravenously.

e) Limitation of the Absorptive Capacity

When the quantity of a substance absorbed does not rise in proportion to an increase in dose, limitation of the absorptive capacity of the intestine must be invoked. This effect is seen with the gastrointestinal absorption of thiamine, β-carotene, amino acids, α-tocopherol and riboflavine. There are no doubt many other substances which are no longer fully absorbed at a certain dosage.

Figure 54 shows a further typical example: after taking ascorbic acid by mouth, the absorbed fraction falls by a mean of $49.5 \pm 4.2\%$ to $16.1 \pm 1.3\%$ when the single dose is increased from 1.5 to 12 g. The invasion curves show that accelerated intestinal passage is not the cause of the reduced absorption.

The doses given therefore give rise to concentrations of substance in the intestinal lumen above the range over which the rate of absorption (v_R) is related linearly to the concentration. The Michaelis-Menten equation of enzyme kinetics and the procedures derived from it may be used in such cases for reactions with a limited rate.

$$v = \frac{v_{max}}{1 + \frac{K}{S}} \quad (79)$$

v, reaction rate
v_{max}, maximal reaction rate
K, Michaelis constant
S, concentration of substance

The dose-dependent processes of absorption described earlier correspond to the extreme of the equation with low concentrations of substance

$$v \rightarrow S \frac{v_{max}}{K} \quad \text{for} \quad K \gg S \quad (79\,a)$$

The invasion constant (k_1) can be substituted for the quotient (v_{max}/K) when the dose administered (D) and the volume of distribution in the body of the substance being studied (V) is substituted in the equation:

$$v_R = \frac{dy_1}{dt} V = D\, k_1 \quad (80)$$

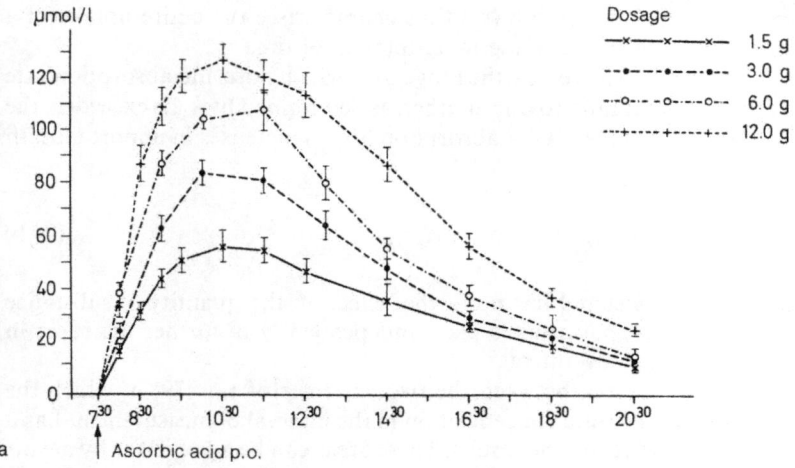
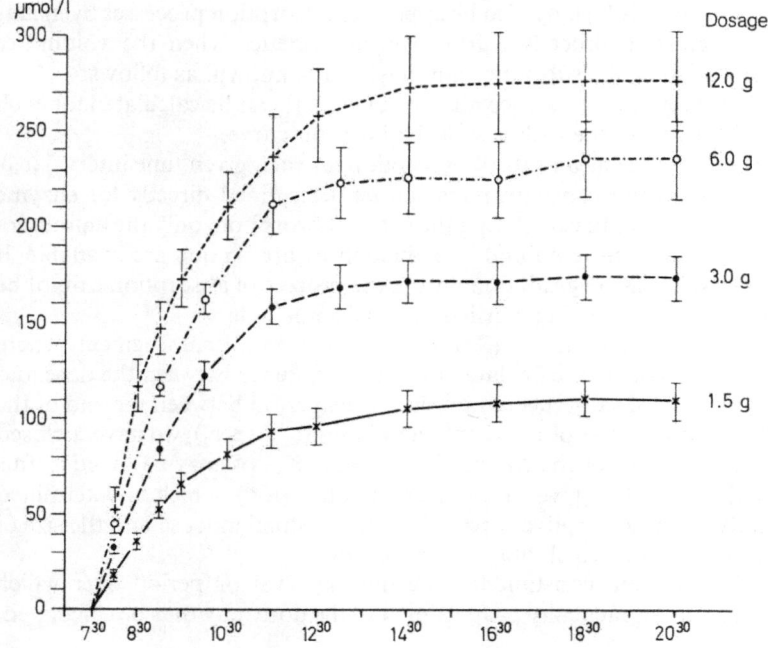

Fig. 54a and b. Absorption of ascorbic acid after different doses. **a** Plasma ascorbic acid. **b** Invasion curves

The rate of absorption (v_R) thus characterises the entire uptake of a substance from the intestine in an interval of time.

If, as the dose increases, the range over which dose and absorption rate are in a constant ratio to one another, as determined by k_1, is exceeded, the limiting value of the rate of absorption ($v_{R_{max}}$) increases in importance. In the extreme case,

$$v \to v_{max} \quad \text{for} \quad S \gg K \tag{79 b}$$

the dose administered has no further effect on the quantity of substance absorbed. Absorption takes place independently of further increases in dose, and at a constant rate.

There is an area between the two extremes of Eq. (79) in which the reduction in substrate concentration in the interval of measurement has a considerable effect on the results. These areas can be allowed for by means of a correction worked out by Ohlenbusch (1965).

By evaluating the invasion curves, the quantities of practical importance from Eq. (79) may also be applied to absorption processes by means of a regression procedure from enzyme kinetics when the volume of distribution of the substance administered is known, as follows:

1. The amount of substance absorbed [$D_{abs}(t)$] can be calculated for each time value from the ordinate of the invasion curve.
2. This gives the mean rate of absorption for each given time interval ($\bar{v}_R$).
3. The substrate concentrations can be determined directly for enzyme kinetics in vitro. In calculating the enteric absorption, only the amount of substance administered and its reduction by absorption are available. If further substrate degradation during the process of absorption cannot be excluded, the following considerations do not hold.

The substrate depot (S^*) lying in the intestinal segment where absorption occurs is calculated from the difference between the dose and the quantity of substance absorbed. In the period between the end of the filling and the start of the emptying phases ($t_1 \leq t \leq t_2$), we have a closed system. In place of the Michaelis constant (K_m) of enzyme kinetics, this calculation in fact gives a complex quantity (K^*), which is determined mainly by the absorptive capacity of the intestinal mucosa and the size of the surface over which absorption occurs.

The invasion constant for the time interval or period over which absorption is practically proportional to the dose may thus be calculated:

$$k_1 = \frac{v_{R_{max}}}{K^*} \tag{81}$$

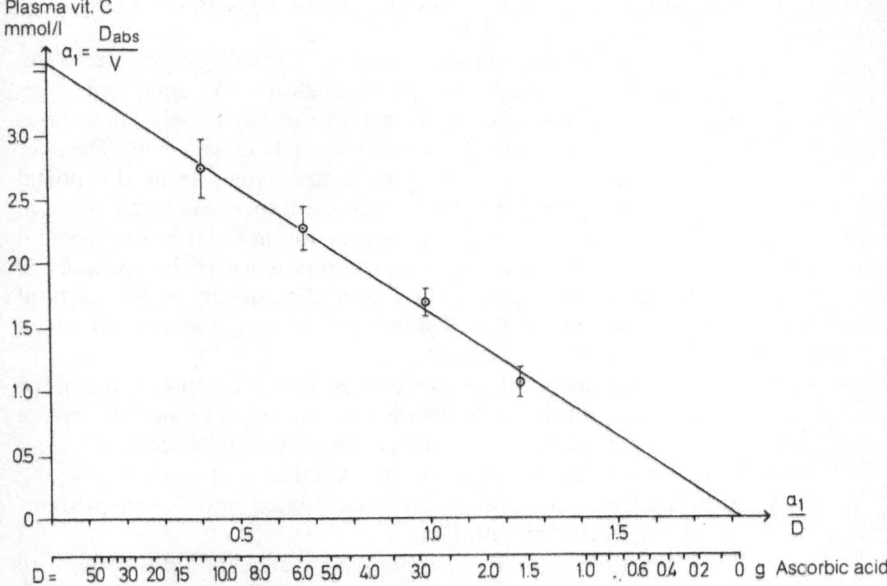

Fig. 55. An estimate of the relation between the dose of ascorbic acid and its absorption. The doses entered on the abscissa are found from the coordinates of the regression lines (y/x)

Using this procedure borrowed from enzyme kinetics, very useful and practical conclusions about the ratio between dose and absorption are obtained from relatively few studies, by varying the dose given (Fig. 55).

f) Different Absorptive Capacity of Two Segments of Intestine

Under the conditions mentioned above, the ratio between the absorbable depot of substance (S^*) and the rate of absorption (v_R) can also be studied at different time intervals in the same process of absorption. For ascorbic acid absorption in healthy adults, we found approximately double the absorption capacity in the proximal as in the distal small intestine (Kübler and Gehler, 1970).

6. Conclusions

a) It is not advisable to apply ready-made formulae schematically in the pharmacokinetic analysis of gastrointestinal absorption, since a multiple but discontinuous system of formulae is involved and numerous unforeseen variants are possible.

b) In addition to the simplest form of virtually complete, dose-dependent absorption which occurs throughout the small intestine, substances can be absorbed preferentially or exclusively in various segments of the gastrointestinal tract (e.g. stomach, distal ileum). The liver can retain substances to a greater or lesser extent from the portal circulation. Invasion may be delayed when substances are transported in the lymphatics. Chemical or physical conversion in the liver or intestinal wall can give rise to invasion curves which in practice are independent of the actual process of absorption. The absorptive capacity of the intestinal mucosa for an unknown range of substances is restricted, a point which must always be taken into account.

c) There are various auxiliary procedures such as reconstruction of the invasion curves, simultaneous loads with substances of known absorptive behaviour, and the study of the time course of urinary excretion.

d) When experimental conditions are suitable, indices such as k_1, t_1, v_{max} and the extent of absorption can be calculated from graphs without the need for elaborate computation.

e) The curves obtained in assessing gastrointestinal absorption are ambiguous to a far greater extent than in other applications of pharmacokinetics, even after all their characteristics have been found. When considered alone, therefore, they cannot *prove* physiological or pharmacological principles, but are quite adequate for the *exclusion* of a hypothesis. Comparative pharmacokinetic studies in man and animals can, therefore, demonstrate where fundamental differences in the metabolic behaviour of drugs and of natural substances occur.

7. Appendix: Some Formulae and Their Derivation

Formulation of the model for gastrointestinal absorption in proportion to the dose.
Invasion curve:

I. $y_1 = a\left(\dfrac{t}{t_1} - \dfrac{1-e^{-k_1 t}}{k_1 t_1}\right)$ for $0 \leqq t \leqq t_1$ (82a)

II. $y_1 = a\left(1 - \dfrac{e^{k_1 t_1}-1}{k_1 t_1} e^{-k_1 t}\right)$ for $t_1 \leqq t \leqq t_2$ (82b)

III. $y_1 = a\left(1 - \dfrac{k_1 t - k_1 t_2 + e^{k_1(t_1+t_2-t)}-1}{k_1 t_1} e^{-k_1 t}\right)$

$$\text{for } t_2 \leq t \leq t_1 + t_2 \quad (82\,c)$$

IV. $y_1 = a(1 - e^{-k_1 t})$ \hfill for $t \geq t_1 + t_2$ \quad (82 d)

Concentration curve:

I. $$y = \frac{a}{k_2 t_1 (k_1 - k_2)} \left(k_1 (1 - e^{-k_2 t}) - k_2 (1 - e^{-k_1 t}) \right)$$

$$\text{for } 0 \leq t \leq t_1 \quad (83\,a)$$

II. $$y = \frac{a}{k_2 t_1 (k_1 - k_2)} \left(k_1 e^{-k_2 t}(e^{k_2 t_1} - 1) - k_2 e^{-k_1 t}(e^{k_1 t_1} - 1) \right)$$

$$\text{for } t_1 \leq t \leq t_2 \quad (83\,b)$$

III. $$y = \frac{a}{k_2 t_1 (k_1 - k_2)} \left(k_1 e^{-k_2 t}(e^{k_2 t_1} + e^{-(k_1 - k_2) t_2} - 1) - k_2 e^{-k_1 (t - t_1)} + \right.$$
$$\left. + (k_1 - k_2) e^{-k_1 t_2} \right) \qquad \textit{for } t_2 \leq t \leq t_1 + t_2 \quad (83\,c)$$

IV. $$y = \frac{a}{k_2 t_1 (k_1 - k_2)} k_1 e^{-k_2 t}(e^{k_2 t_1} - 1)(1 - e^{-(k_1 - k_2) t_2})$$

$$\text{for } t \geq t_1 + t_2 \quad (83\,d)$$

Secondary depot after absorption in proportion to the dose.
Invasion curve:

I. $$y_1 = \frac{k_{121}}{k_{12}} \frac{a}{(k_{11} - k_{12}) t_1} \left((k_{11} - k_{12}) t + \frac{k_1}{k_{11}} (1 - e^{-k_{11} t}) + \right.$$
$$\left. - \frac{k_{11}}{k_{12}} (1 - e^{-k_{12} t}) \right) \qquad \text{for } 0 \leq t \leq t_1 \quad (84\,a)$$

II. $$y_1 = \frac{k_{121}}{k_{12}} \frac{a}{(k_{11} - k_{12}) t_1} \left((k_{11} - k_{12}) t_1 + \frac{k_{12}}{k_{11}} (e^{k_{11} t_1} - 1) e^{-k_{11} t} + \right.$$
$$\left. - \frac{k_{11}}{k_{12}} (e^{k_{12} t_1} - 1) e^{-k_{12} t} \right) \qquad \text{for } t_1 \leq t \leq t_2 \quad (84\,b)$$

III. $$y_1 = \frac{k_{121}}{k_{12}} \frac{a}{(k_{11} - k_{12}) t_1} \left((k_{11} - k_{12}) t_1 - (k_{11} - k_{12})(t - t_2) e^{-k_{11} t_2} + \right.$$
$$+ \frac{k_{12}}{k_{11}} (e^{-k_{11}(t - t_1)} - e^{-k_{11} t_2}) + \frac{k_{11}}{k_{12}} e^{-k_{11} t_2} (1 - e^{-k_{12}(t - t_2)}) +$$
$$\left. - \frac{k_{11}}{k_{12}} (e^{k_{12} \cdot t_1} - 1) e^{-k_{12} t} \right) \qquad \text{for } t_2 \leq t \leq t_1 + t_2 \quad (84\,c)$$

IV. $y_1 = \dfrac{k_{121}}{k_{12}} \dfrac{a}{(k_{11}-k_{12})t_1} ((k_{11}-k_{122})(1-e^{-k_{11}t_2})t_1 +$

$\qquad - \dfrac{k_{11}}{k_{12}} (1-e^{-(k_{11}-k_{12})t_2})(e^{k_{12}t_1}-1)e^{-k_{12}t})$

$\hfill \text{for} \quad t \geq t_1 + t_2 \qquad (84\,\text{d})$

Derivation of invasion curves—reconstruction

$$\frac{dy}{dt} = \frac{dy_1}{dt} - k_2 y$$

can be transformed as

$$dy_1 = dy + k_2 y \, dt$$

By integration,

$$y_1(t) = y(t) + k_2 \int_0^t y \, dt \qquad (73)$$

Derivation of the procedure for determining t_1.
Penetration phase (II) of the invasion curve:

II. $y_1 = a\left(1 - \dfrac{e^{k_1 t_1}-1}{k_1 t_1} e^{-k_1 t}\right) \qquad \text{for} \quad t_1 \leq t \leq t_2 \qquad (82\,\text{b})$

$y_1 = a(1 - C e^{-k_1 t})$, when

$$C = \frac{e^{k_1 t_1}-1}{k_1 t_1} \qquad (77)$$

VIII. Interaction

Pharmacokinetic indices should be regarded as standard biological quantities. A given substance always yields the same values in the same subjects under the same conditions. This behaviour enables organ function tests to be evaluated and dosage to be calculated, especially for repetitive and long-term therapy.

The standard pharmacokinetic values may be affected by a number of factors, however, sometimes to a considerable degree. It is very important to know about these factors and to take them into account in calculating dosage and in evaluating function tests. The intentional manipulation of such parameters can also be valuable in allowing exogenous or endogenous poisons to be eliminated more rapidly.

The influence of various factors on pharmacokinetics in general and on the individual pharmacokinetic indices for exogenous and endogenous substances in particular should be dealt with collectively under the heading of interaction. This ability to affect the elimination rate is of great interest, although the inconstancy of the size of the distribution volume must also be borne in mind.

1. Elimination

a) Pathological Changes in the Organ of Excretion

Pathological changes can sometimes impair the function of an organ considerably. Tests of function using suitable test substances give much information about the residual functional capacity of the organ during the course of a disease and by comparison with healthy subjects. It is immaterial whether the volume clearance (in the classical sense of van Slyke), the time clearance (half-time method of Dost), the isotope technique, or the considerably less comprehensive retention test or excretion sample are used. In every case the excretory capacity and ultimately the rate of elimination are determined, or at least play a considerable part in the result.

Since a delay in the elimination of a test substance indicates disease in the organ which plays the major part in its excretion, all drugs excreted by that organ will be eliminated more slowly in affected patients.

Thus a pathological bromsulphalein test or intravenous bilirubin load indicates hepatocellular disease, in which case drugs excreted or metabolised predominantly by the liver, such as phenylbutazone, steroids, salicylates, n-acetylaminophenol, azorubin, para-aminobenzoic acid, chloramphenicol and sulphonamides, would also be eliminated more slowly.

In a similar way, inulin, creatinine and thiosulphate indicate disorders of glomerular filtration which would affect the excretion of such drugs as streptomycin, isoniazid, tetracycline, ethambutol and cephaloridine.

Disorders of renal function or of total renal excretory function are demonstrated by using phenol red or PAH. Here, too, the degree of retardation of elimination correlates very well with the extent of the functional disorder in the organ. A number of drugs act in the same way as the test substance, including penicillin and its semi-synthetic derivatives, cephalothin, nitrofurantoin, and contrast media for the radiological demonstration of the efferent urinary tract.

Where excretion is inadequate, as when a drug normally excreted by the kidneys is given to a patient with renal failure, its repeated administration leads to accumulation if the impaired organ function is not taken into account when calculating dosage. Such disorders can nowadays be quantitated and compensated for with the aid of pharmacokinetics. The principle involved is simple to understand and to put into practice.

The mean concentration of a drug in the steady state during continuous therapy ($\bar{y}^*$) is directly proportional to the dose per unit time ($\dot{D}$) and inversely proportional to the total clearance of the substance concerned which is the sum of renal and extrarenal (i.e. metabolic or hepatic) clearances:

$$\bar{y}^* = \frac{\dot{D}}{Cl_{ren} + Cl_{n\text{-}ren}} \tag{85}$$

In uraemic subjects for the renally excreted fraction of a drug, the endogenous creatinine clearance appears to be proportional to the renal clearance and so, provided the proportionality factor (f) can be found, the equation $\bar{y}^* = \dfrac{\dot{D}}{f \cdot Cl_{creat} + Cl_{n\text{-}ren}}$ can be applied to individual drugs.

b) Age-Dependent Changes in Elimination

Most substances studied to date are excreted much more slowly in the neonate than in older children. This is probably in part due to the fact that many enzymes necessary for detoxication have very little activity in the liver cells of the newborn. These enzymatic functions do not mature fully until after the first few weeks or months of life. This applies in addition to the test substance bromsulphalein (Fig. 56), to bilirubin and to the appropriate drugs mentioned in the previous section.

Studies with indocyanine green have shown that the carrier protein which transports this test substance through the liver cell is deficient in the neonate. Indocyanine green is therefore eliminated much more slowly in the neonate than in the older child.

Glomerular filtration and *tubular secretion* are also impaired in the newborn, however, as shown by studies with inulin, thiosulphate, PAH and phenol red, and this of course also affects the analogous drugs mentioned in the previous section. This functional immaturity may be due to the fact that, although the neonatal kidney possesses its full complement of nephrons, all are not fully included in the circulation until after the first period of life. Ultramicroscopic differences are also seen in the basement membranes of the glomerular loops, which are initially thicker and three-layered, but later thinner and two-layered.

From the age of 6 months to about 2 years, a few drugs such as sulphonamides appear to be eliminated more rapidly than in older children or adults. Some studies substantiate a shortening of the half-time of elimination by one-fifth to one-quarter in comparison with the norm for adults. Here, too, there are consequences for treatment, such as the need to raise the dose or shorten the dose interval.

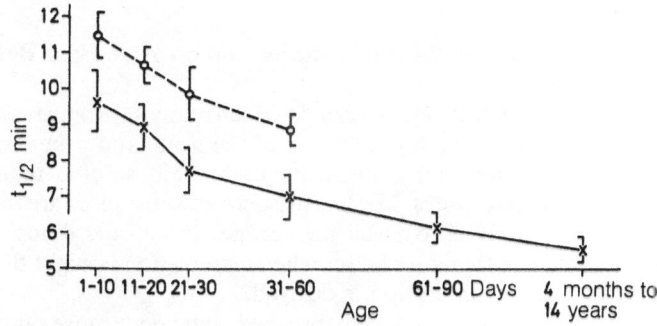

Fig. 56. The half-time of elimination of bromsulphalein in relation to age

Delayed elimination is also seen in the elderly. All studies to date show such a great scatter, however, that it seems pointless to quote calculable or predictable values.

The amount of damage incurred throughout life, together with involutionary changes, which vary greatly from individual to individual, will inevitably necessitate the basing of future therapeutic regimens and dosage corrections on concentrations of active substance. Renal function appears to deteriorate before hepatic, and the wheel appears to have turned full circle from childhood to old age. At all events, when treating the child up to 3 months of age or the elderly person, the effects described must be taken into account.

c) Pharmacogenetic Factors

Only two details need mentioning under the heading of pharmaco*genetics*. Inborn errors of metabolism are rare and are either discovered early during screening tests or manifest themselves in functional disturbances which may require investigation and long-term treatment in special centres. We may quote the example of glucuronyl transferase deficiency, where not only is bilirubin conjugation inhibited but glucuronidation is also affected, and hence the elimination of many drugs. Other diseases in this group have no marked effect on pharmacokinetics.

One situation has reinforced the concept of pharmacogenetics, namely that the rate of elimination of a number of substances is obviously genetically determined and varies within individual ethnic groups. The elimination of isonicotinic acid hydrazide has been studied in detail. 'Slow inactivators' with a half-time of elimination of about 160 min and 'rapid inactivators' with a half-time of elimination of 60 min have been found. Further studies are necessary.

d) Dependence of Rate of Elimination on Acid-Base Balance

One factor which affects the rate at which many substances are eliminated is the hydrogen ion concentration of the urine and other body fluids.

Undissociated compounds are more lipid soluble than ionised or highly dissociated ones. The less dissociated substances are thus transported more readily across cell membranes (non-ionic diffusion). Tubular reabsorption is therefore better when dissociation is slight than when it is greater and so elimination is delayed.

Weak acids are less well reabsorbed, and hence more rapidly excreted, in alkaline than in acid urine, since they are more highly ionised in an alkaline than in an acid medium. Weak bases, on the other hand, are more rapidly excreted in acid urine. For the same reasons, alkaloids such as morphine and its derivatives appear in acid gastric juice.

This behaviour is important in situations such as septicaemia, prolonged attacks of fever, gastroenteritis, intoxication and respiratory acidosis, in all of which the urine is almost invariably acid. The buffering of decompensated acidosis on the other hand, produces an alkaline urine. Considerable changes in the rate of elimination of a drug can result.

Alkalinisation can bring about a threefold increase in the rate of elimination of a sulphonamide. Severe infantile dyspepsia or gastroenteritis can greatly retard the elimination of various sulphonamides in the acute phase when compared with convalescence. The circadian rhythm of acid-base balance is associated with parallel changes in the rate of elimination of sulphonamides and amphetamines during the day. Disorders of acid-base balance have been associated during long-term therapy with up to tenfold deviations from the expected concentrations, an astonishing discrepancy. Therapeutic use may be made of this effect in the treatment of poisoning. Alkalinisation of the urine in barbiturate overdosage and acidification and removal of the acid gastric juice in morphine and codeine poisoning is part of the modern treatment of such mishaps. It is nevertheless still not usual to consider acid-base balance when calculating dosage regimens routinely.

Table 5. Excretion of weak acids and weak bases in alkaline and acid urine, respectively. More rapid elimination in:

Alkaline urine	Acid urine
Sulphonamides	Amphetamine
Salicylates	Mepacrine
PAH	Chloroquine
Phenobarbitone	Santoquine
Barbitone	Nicotine
Phenylbutazone	Quinine
Citric acid	Procaine
p-Aminobenzoic acid	5-Hydroxytryptamine
Probenecid	Pethidine
Indolacetic acid	Dexamphetamine
Phenol red	Adrenaline
Bromcresol green	Levorphanol
Bromphenol blue	Morphine
2,4-Dinitrophenol	Codeine
Nitrofurantoin	
Carbutamide	
Amino acids	

Table 5 lists some weak acids, which are therefore excreted more slowly in acid than in alkaline urine, and contrasts them with some weak bases which pass more rapidly into alkaline urine.

e) Circadian Rhythm of Excretion Rate

The circadian rhythms in excretion rate found up to now have involved sulphonamides and have been easily explained in terms of the rhythm of acid-base balance. The slight nocturnal acidosis retards the excretion of the weakly acid sulphonamides during the night more than by day.

The circadian variations in serum iron concentration occasioned an investigation of the biokinetic behaviour of this metabolite. These studies showed that the daily rhythmic variations in serum iron concentration are due predominantly to variations in the size of the endogenous input, that is, the metabolic transfer. Variations in the half-time of elimination, (turnover rate) have a slight effect. A study of other endogenous substances should shed more light on this problem.

f) Water Diuresis and Rate of Elimination

A further, active means of affecting the elimination process is to modify the renal excretion of a substance by accelerating the flow of urine. This idea is based on limiting the time available for tubular reabsorption by means of a water diuresis, thereby accelerating the rate of excretion. Very large quantities of fluid are necessary to achieve such an effect. A true forced diuresis in adults is associated with urine volumes of at least 500–800 ml/h, i.e. 12–20 litres in 24 h. Smaller volumes have no effect. Even such high volumes cannot bring about glycosuria, although tubular reabsorption also prevents glucose excretion by the kidney.

Elimination rates can therefore only be modified to any significant extent by very high volumes of fluid.

g) Solvent Deficiency

One observation, which relates more to electrolyte balance than to pharmacokinetics, is worthy of note here. Healthy adults can tolerate very large supplementary salt loads (30 g/day) so long as their fluid intake is unrestricted. Fluid restriction limits salt excretion. Restriction of water limited salt elimination. Sodium is retained together with water and the extracellular fluid space expanded as a result.

This situation is one of severe solvent deficiency. These experiments have been reproduced in infants in that some antidiarrhoeal diets which have been widely used in the past had such a high mineral content that, over a period of time, they caused an increase in weight due to sodium and fluid retention. By giving fluid supplementation, sodium could be eliminated, the extracellular fluid space returned to normal and the body weight reduced.

The renal clearance of many substances is also reduced in severe dehydration, another form of solvent deficiency, although haemodynamic factors also play a part here.

The intake of large doses of poorly soluble sulphonamides in the past has led to crystalluria and very severe renal damage. Sulphonamides of this nature are no longer used. An unfavourable acid-base balance and a relative solvent deficiency led to a crystallisation in the tubular urine of the substances themselves and of their metabolites.

Conditions of water loss, as well as of overload with the substance to be eliminated, can therefore retard the rate of elimination. Precipitation in the efferent urinary tract should nowadays be extremely rare, however.

h) Enzyme Induction

Interest has recently been aroused in another principle by which foreign substances are actively and more rapidly eliminated from the body, namely that of enzyme induction. More than 200 substances with this effect have been described to date. They bring about an increase in the number of organelles in the liver cells where enzymes responsible for drug elimination by demethylation, conjugation or oxidation are localised.

The best known of these substances are barbiturates, glutethimide, tolbutamide, nikethamide, a few oncogenic agents and insecticides. The effects of phenobarbitone have been extensively studied and our group has worked on the xanthine derivative, xanthinolnicotinate. These substances bring about an obvious increase in the membranes of the smooth endoplasmic reticulum which is associated with increased enzymatic activity as seen both in vitro and in vivo, where the rate of elimination of a whole series of substances is increased.

Enzyme induction is therefore of great practical importance. It leads to faster metabolism and hence faster excretion of drugs, so the concentration of active substance in the body falls below the effective level earlier than would otherwise occur. Calculations of dosage and dose interval are no longer accurate when the substance is given to pretreated volunteers in whom enzymes have been induced. The possibility of the occurrence of such a phenomenon should always be borne in mind when using drug combinations.

Anticoagulant therapy may be affected when the dosage is adjusted on the basis of coagulation studies. Dicoumarol anticoagulants are more rapidly excreted in patients taking phenobarbitone at the same time, and so need to be given in higher doses. When the phenobarbitone is stopped, however, the dicoumarol is eliminated more slowly again and may accumulate, often leading in the patient to a dangerous tendency to bleed.

In paediatrics, enzyme induction can be particularly important in the newborn. Many substances are metabolised much more slowly in the first 3 months of life than in older children. This functional impairment is due to the very low activity of a number of enzymes which only achieve their full function gradually during maturation.

The more rapid elimination of test substances and drugs by an opposing mechanism is of academic interest only if one knows the elimination data for the age in question and takes these into account in diagnosis and therapy. Bilirubin, however, is a substance which is metabolised by enzymes from the microsomal fraction and the endoplasmic reticulum to a form capable of being eliminated. Bilirubin is formed when haemoglobin is broken down and also (as 'shunt bilirubin') in haemoglobin synthesis. Glucuronyl transferase is one of the enzyme group which shows very low activity in the neonate, only maturing slowly to reach full function after the first few weeks of life. This enzyme glucuronidates bilirubin to a form which can be excreted. Depending on how well the system for glucuronidation functions in the post-partum period, a certain degree of jaundice (icterus neonatorum) due to retarded bilirubin excretion arises which can be further intensified by an increase in endogenous production (haemolysis, haematoma, toxic or septic processes).

Unconjugated bilirubin is normally transported bound to albumin. If the serum concentration is very high and the binding capacity of the albumin exceeded, the excess bilirubin can penetrate the cells of the cerebral nuclei where it has a toxic effect by uncoupling oxidative phosphorylation, so giving rise to the clinical disease of kernicterus. Acceleration of bilirubin elimination by enzyme induction would appear to be a worthwhile measure. The results from animal experiments, however, have varied with different species and experimental procedures, suggesting that one should not extrapolate too readily from the small laboratory animal to man. Such animal experiments do, on the other hand, give us the opportunity to test the applicability of the principle of enzyme induction to practical medicine.

Several investigators reported the successful use of phenobarbitone in cases of Crigler–Najjar syndrome. By using phenobarbitone, the bilirubin excretion in these cases of congenital glucuronyl transferase deficiency was increased so much that the initially high blood concentrations of bilirubin soon fell to much lower levels. When the barbiturate was stopped, the bilirubin increased once more. Experiments with salicylamide showed that the capacity for glucuronidation actually increased. This effect of phenobarbitone was reproducible on many occasions.

By pre-treating experimental animals with phenobarbitone a definite increase in the rate of bilirubin elimination can be achieved. Treatment of the mother animals until delivery resulted in definite enzyme induction in the newborn. A few investigators have been able to achieve a regular reduction in the serum bilirubin concentration in young infants by giving phenobarbitone in the first few days of life, whereas other groups have not observed this effect.

We studied the effect of phenobarbitone on the rate of elimination of sulphasomidine. Since pilot experiments showed the most marked changes to be a few days after a 3-day course of barbiturates, we gave patients intramuscular phenobarbitone once a day for 3 days in doses between 10 and 20 mg/kg. The half-time of elimination of sulphasomidine was estimated beforehand, on the third day after stopping the barbiturate and a few days later (Table 6).

Phenobarbitone has a similar effect on the elimination of bromsulphalein, just as does the xanthine derivative xanthinolnicotinate, which increases the rate of elimination of both sulphasomidine and bromsulphalein (Table 6).

Table 6. Half-time of elimination of sulphasomidine and bromsulphalein before and after treatment with phenobarbitone and xanthinolnicotinate

	No.	Age	$t_{50\%}$		
			Before	After 3 days treatment	3 days after treatment
Experiment with phenobarbitone (20 mg/kg/d)					
Sulphasomidine	21	1.6 mo	7.0 h	6.0 h	5.1 h
Bromsulphalein	12	2.7 mo	9.6 min	9.4 min	7.4 min
Experiment with xanthinolnicotinate (60–100 mg/kg/d)					
Sulphasomidine	23	12 d	15.0 h	10.2 h	
Bromsulphalein	6	22 d	11.0 min	10.4 min	8.5 min

Table 7

Phenobarbitone treatment (7.5 mg/kg/d)	Neonates $n=10$	Maximal rate of elimination, V_{max} $\mu Mol \cdot l^{-1} \cdot min$
Indocyanine green elimination		Before Treatment After
		45 63

We were finally able to show that giving phenobarbitone clearly reduces the bilirubin concentration in comparison with untreated children.

It is not only the microsomal liver enzymes but also the transport proteins in the liver cell which appear to be inducible by phenobarbitone. Studies with indocyanine green have shown this dyestuff to be bound to transport proteins in the liver cell in the course of its selective uptake. Elimination of the dye from the blood obeys saturation kinetics. The maximum rate of elimination, V_{max}, can be clearly increased by treating with phenobarbitone (Table 7).

Further studies are needed to show how effective enzyme induction can be in the routine treatment of metabolic hyperbilirubinaemia and in other clinical conditions such as poisoning, for example. When treating with more than one drug simultaneously or sequentially, however, the possibility of one drug inducing enzymes which can accelerate the elimination of another must always be borne in mind.

i) Inhibition of Elimination by Toxicity

When given in doses which can cause toxicity, a few drugs can inhibit their own elimination. Such effects are really aspects of toxicology or pharmacology. The reactions involved on pharmacokinetics, of damage to individual organs and their function, are the same as those discussed in Section 1.a. of this chapter.

α) Displacement from Protein Binding

A large fraction of both exogenous and endogenous substances is generally transported in the blood bound to protein, and particularly to albumin. This vehicular function of albumin is of course stoichiometrically limited. The binding and the ratio of the bound to the non-bound fraction of the substance concerned obey the law of mass action. Here, however, the actual relationships between the free, bound and total fractions vary greatly from substance to substance.

The affinity of individual substances is, moreover, different, so that some substances can displace others from their protein-binding sites. Thus sulphonamides can displace bilirubin from its albumin binding, releasing it prematurely from the blood into the tissues to cause, in the neonate, kernicterus, even at lower bilirubin concentrations than would otherwise be considered a risk.

On the other hand, when the binding capacity of protein-bound drugs is exceeded, excretion becomes more rapid and complex curves arise which can only be interpreted pharmacokinetically when this mechanism is taken into account in the calculation.

Apart from neonatal jaundice with its danger of kernicterus, exceeding the binding capacity and displacement from protein-binding sites is rarely of importance, since drug doses of the necessary order of magnitude are not usual.

β) Clearance Depression

A further factor to affect elimination is clearance depression. The capacity of the kidneys for tubular secretion is limited. When several substances excreted by this route are given at the same time, therefore, they may each be excreted more slowly than usual. Such an effect is found when PAH clearances are measured during high-dosage penicillin therapy. A similar fluctuant effect is also seen with cephalothin, nitrofurantoin, diodon (an X-ray contrast medium) and caronamide (a sulphonamide). Obviously when one of these substances alone exceeds the tubular capacity, a situation like that known as self-depression of clearance can arise. Thus exceeding a serum PAH concentration of 50–100 mg/litre can give rise to clearance values which are not truly representative of renal function (*cf*. Sect. III. e).

γ) Acceleration of Elimination by Chelating Agents and Adsorbants Given Orally

A form of reciprocal action is mentioned here which has recently come to our notice. Doxycycline, a tetracycline with an apparently long half-time of elimination which it achives by its high degree of gastrointestinal reabsorption, forms chelates with iron compounds which are virtually not absorbed. When iron and doxycycline are given at the same time, chelates are formed, as a result of which doxycycline is eliminated much more rapidly. A number of adsorbants commonly prescribed in gastroenteritis have a similar effect, adsorbing an antibiotic given orally at the same time and thereby preventing its absorption by the body. Ion exchange resins also act similarly.

2. Volume of Distribution

a) Hydration and Dehydration

Disorders of water balance frequently result in changes in the size of the fluid space, often long before signs of decompensation are seen. Considerable variation in the volume of the extracellular fluid reservoir can occur. Since this space determines, or is involved in, the distribution volume of many drugs, variations in drug concentration caused thereby must be taken into account. The great capacity for water uptake by structures in the child's interstitial tissues and the greater hydrolability of the child's body are also important in this context.

The extracellular fluid volume can increase in infants to 170% of the norm without visible oedema, and can fall to 56% of its normal value. Such changes have never been seen in adults without oedema or severe signs of decompensation. If the volume of distribution of a drug and the size of the extracellular fluid space are the same, and a drug concentration of, say, 100 mg/litre could be achieved in a healthy child, then the concentration in a child with a water load given the same dose would be 59 mg/litre and in the dehydrated child, 230 mg/litre.

Such extreme values are rare, but more moderate variations are relatively frequent. With changes of about 20% in the volume of distribution, the resultant concentration-time curves for a drug whose rates of absorption and elimination are constant are shown in Fig. 57. The

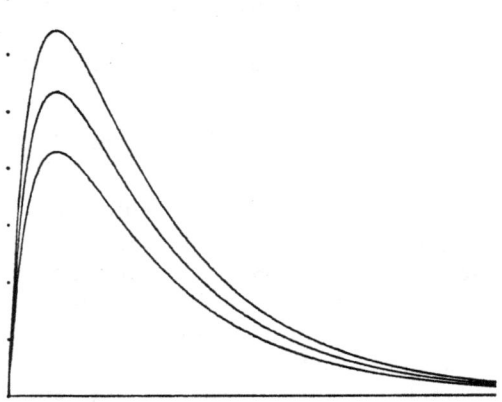

Fig. 57. Concentration-time curves with changing volumes of distribution. Middle curve: reference curve. Upper curve: volume of distribution 20% lower. Lower curve: volume of distribution 20% higher

overall ratio of the concentrations is 12 : 10 : 8. Such variations for different drugs must influence the effectiveness of treatment, especially when the dose is only roughly estimated.

We should also remember that changes of this order in the size of the extracellular fluid space can be brought about by a single dose of a saluretic or infusion of a salt-containing fluid.

b) Hydropic States

Hydropic states such as hydrocephalus, ascites or hydrothorax considerably increase the volume of distribution for a number of drugs. Inclusion of fluid collections of this nature in calculations of dosage is made more difficult by the fact that they do not undergo the rapid mixing and turnover found in physiological spaces.

In infants with hydrocephalus or patients with severe ascites, for example, a single intravenous injection of a test substance does not give rise to elimination curves which are capable of mathematical or pharmacokinetic assessment, and a steady state is only obtained after a long delay during continuous infusion.

These conditions are very unclear and the issue is not clarified by drainage, dehydration experiments, etc.; therefore they are only mentioned here.

3. Conclusions

Terms such as synergism, addition and antagonism are purely pharmacological, and have nothing to do with the pharmacokinetic concept of interaction.

Interaction, or the effects of the pharmacokinetic parameters for exogenous and endogenous substances, can be brought about by very different factors which must be included in calculations of dosage and the evaluation of function tests. An interaction may result not only in high concentrations in the toxic range but also in lack of effect due to too small a concentration of the drug.

The side-effects of toxic concentrations are generally dealt with promptly by appropriate measures when they first appear. The side-effects of underdosage, on the other hand, are much less obvious although they occur much more commonly than is generally realised, and are potentially just as serious, if not more so.

For all that, it is true to say that we are still only at a very early stage in the study of factors which can cause interaction.

IX. Use of Analogue Computers in Pharmacokinetics

The development of computer technology in recent years has brought substantial advantages to almost every field of science. Where detailed observations can be analysed automatically, the investigator has more time to plan and carry out experiments. Experimental results can now be analysed mathematically by computer where they would have been a great burden to a biological scientist with no special training in mathematics. The use of computers has not only lightened our work-load, however; it has also enhanced our knowledge of laws and relationships in nature and has opened up new methods and areas of work which can then be thoroughly investigated by the classic experimental procedures. However, the lightening of the work-load in data processing is more than outweighed by the new tasks to which it gives rise.

The word 'computer' usually conjures up an image of a large machine which adds, subtracts, multiplies and divides with unbelievable rapidity and is able to draw comparisons and even make decisions. Such machines are generally digital computers. A digital computer in fact merely adds and subtracts. Multiplication is achieved by repeated additions, and comparisons by establishing whether a sum is zero or not zero.

In the digital computer, we must be able to express the computational quantity, that is, the quantity which is to be changed by algebraic operations, as a pattern of individual 'yes-no' situations. An experimental value is modified by changing this pattern, that is, by changing the individual 'yes-no' situations in sequence. The task of undertaking such a change must in turn be generated by a number of such 'yes-no' patterns. Each computer operation, therefore, has to be subdivided into a series of successive steps whose intermediate results must be retained. A digital computer calculates like a child who uses his fingers to help him add 2 to 3, since his memory is not yet able to retain the intermediate results, i.e. the 3 and the 4.

These apparent disadvantages are compensated for by the great speed with which a digital computer performs each basic operation, and by the fact that the machine has access to an almost unlimited storage capacity for the uptake of data, intermediate results and programme steps.

A real disadvantage for the experimental scientist, however, is the labour of programming which, notwithstanding the development of 'problem-orientated' computer languages, must be left to specialists. The validity of different pharmacokinetic models cannot, therefore, be tested by this means without the support of at least a computer programmer, if not a mathematician. The models must, moreover, be set out as explicit equations.

The analogue computer, on the other hand, meets the requirements of the experimental scientist much better. Programming is simple, needs little time, and programmes can be rapidly changed. The execution of a programme can be monitored on a screen and continuously interpreted. The protocol of the programme is expressed graphically and each user can see his own problems displayed in it without needing translation into a programmable language. The requirement for programming is not so much mathematics as the ability to think in models and to have some understanding of technical processes. A certain aptitude for creative handwork can also be very helpful.

1. Principle of the Analogue Computer

In order to grasp the principle by which analogue computers work, one must understand that many different processes in nature can be expressed by the same mathematical formula. For example, the equation for the concentration changes in the blood with time of a drug given intramuscularly is identical with that formulated by Bateman to describe the natural decay of a radioactive substance into further labile daughter

Table 8. Constants analogous with the pharmacokinetic constant k_{ij} from other special fields. Acknowledgement to Dost, F. H., *Grundlagen der Pharmakokinetik* (1968)

Constant analogous with k_{ij}	Speciality
Rate constant of elimination	Pharmacokinetics
Coefficient of clearance	Nephrology
Decay constant	Nuclear physics
Absorption constant	Optics
Coefficient of friction	Mechanics
Reciprocal time constant	Electricity
Coefficient of self-induction	Electricity
Birth rate	Population statistics
Mortality	Population statistics
Logarithmic coefficient of regression	Mathematics
Decrement (increment) of geometrical series	Mathematics

elements. The coefficient of transfer of a substance in pharmacokinetics and the decay constant of nuclear physics are analogous in the same way as are the amounts of an isotope and a drug in a compartment.

Constants analogous with k_2 and drawn from various fields of natural science are summarised in Table 8. We may conclude from this table that each process in one of these specialities has a mathematical counterpart in other fields. The analogue computer is based on this principle.

Anyone wishing to investigate the regularity of a pharmacokinetic model could do so by constructing an electrical circuit which can be described by the same mathematical formula as the model in which he is interested. This circuit is then an analogue computer programme.

The computational quantity in the analogue computer is the electrical potential difference, which is measured in volts. This potential difference is subjected in the electrical circuit to electrophysical processes analogous to those which affect the concentration in the biological situation. The independent variable is always time, measured in seconds.

The computer operations take place in electronic modules, of which there are three important types:
1) *Operational amplifiers*, which deliver at their output the sum of the voltages presented at their input with signs reversed and amplified if required by a factor of 10. The amplifiers are arranged in such a way as to protect the voltage at the output from being reduced by the additional load of further computing components. Thus changes are brought about only by intentional computing operations.
2) *Capacitors*, which are integrating elements. They can be used only when connected to amplifiers at whose output, consequently, the integral with respect to time of the sum of the inputs, again with signs reversed, is available.
3) *Coefficient potentiometers* are regarded as passive elements. By adjusting these resistors manually until a desired conductance is obtained, the analogous computational quantity can be multiplied by a factor between 0 and 1.

There are other modules which multiply two time-dependent values, or which enable two variables to be compared. Special functions such as logarithms, sinus functions and others can also be provided.

The terminals for the inputs and outputs of all the computing elements are set out on an interchangeable *plugboard* or patch panel where they can be interconnected as required by plugs and wires to construct a programme. The voltage changes in any element can be displayed from here as required on an oscillograph or an x–y plotter.

Thus an analogue computer is like a box of bricks which contains the functions of reversal of sign, addition, multiplication and the integral with

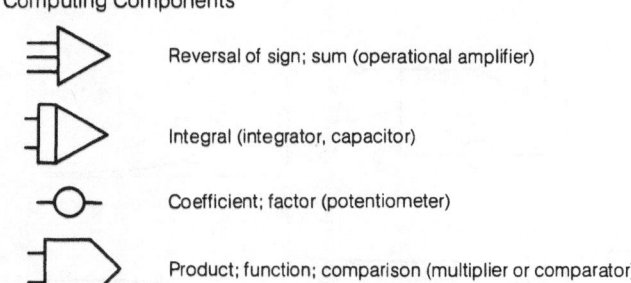

Fig. 58. Symbols used in the display of computer operations in an analogue computer programme

time as its building bricks. The computer programme is displayed in the form of a circuit diagram as a combination of these building bricks. For this purpose, the individual components are denoted by certain, generally agreed symbols (Fig. 58).

2. Programming the Analogue Computer

A capacitor behaves like a pharmacokinetic compartment. When it is brought to a certain potential and then short-circuited over a resistance, the charge and hence also the voltage always falls in unit time by the same fraction in exactly the same way as the amount of drug in a compartment.

The analogous circuit for a first-order compartment therefore consists of an integrator (capacitor with amplifier), for which the input and output are connected through a feedback potentiometer. If one wishes to describe the events which follow a single injection, the capacitor must be brought to the starting voltage which corresponds to the dose (IC, initial condition) (Fig. 59, *upper part*) before the calculation can begin. To simulate continuous infusion, the voltage corresponding to the infusion rate is applied to one of the inputs throughout the calculation (Fig. 59, *lower part*). The two cases are distinguished from one another only by the choice of one of two sockets. The rate constant of elimination, k_2, is given by the conductance of the feedback potentiometer.

In this brief account, an analogue computer programme to study a one-compartment system has already been presented without, surprisingly, any need for mathematical formulae. It has been sufficient to apply known models.

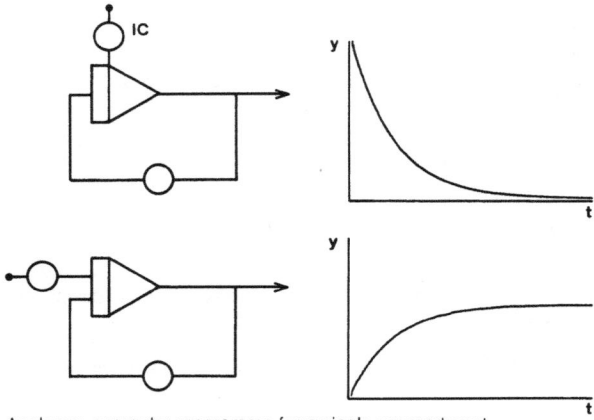

Analogue computer programme for a single compartment

Fig. 59. Representation of a one-compartment pharmacokinetic model as an analogue computer programme (for symbols, see Fig. 58). The computer results are shown as a concentration-time curve next to the circuit diagram.
Upper figure: single injection. Before the computer cycle begins, the integrator is brought to the voltage corresponding to the initial dose (IC, initial condition).
Lower figure: continuous infusion. The voltage corresponding to the infusion rate is applied to the input throughout the period of the computer operation. The conductance of the potentiometer linking the input and output corresponds to the rate constant of elimination, k_{20}

Some simple algebraic symbols are nevertheless useful in preserving this broad view when considering the effects in several compartments. This is where the analogue computer shows its particular advantage. Since the integral is directly available as a building block, it is enough to write down separately the rates of change, i.e. the differential equations for the individual compartments, and then to assign an integrator to each compartment.

This procedure is shown in Fig. 60 as an example of the Bateman function: the box diagram can be expressed as a system of differential equations whose initial conditions are a dose D at time $t = 0$ present entirely in the muscle depot and a blood concentration of the drug of zero. The blood concentration y is determined by the quantity of drug B and the volume of distribution V.

There are therefore two integrators in the programme at whose inputs the conditions of the individual equations are fulfilled. The quantities M and B are given reversed signs by this procedure. It now becomes possible to incorporate further compartments (integrators) without difficulty, and to take several rate constants into account, as occurs in reversible processes.

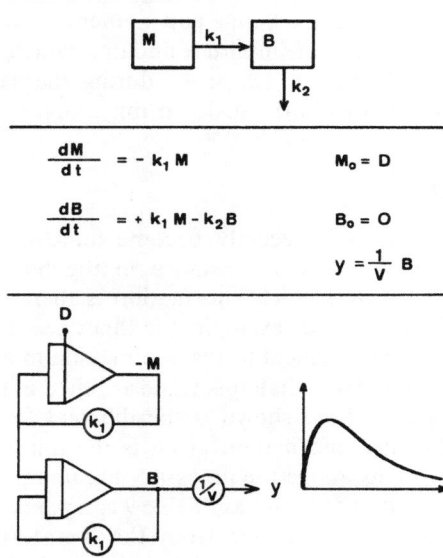

Fig. 60. The Bateman function used to describe the blood concentration-time curve after a single intramuscular injection of a drug. The four identical forms of representation, namely a box diagram, a system of differential equations, a programme expressed as a circuit diagram, and a graph of the time curve for one compartment, show the series of steps by which the analogue computer can be used to take a problem through from its inception to its solution. M, drug concentration in the intramuscular depot; D, dose; B, amount of drug in the blood; V, volume of distribution; y, blood concentration; k_{12}, invasion constant; k_{20}, elimination constant

This illustration contains the four aspects of a pharmacokinetic model as seen by an analogue computer user, namely the box diagram, the system of differential equations, the programme represented as a circuit diagram and the graph of the curve for one compartment. The explicit equation for the e-functions plays no part in this.

In order to be able to compute numerically, a further property must be taken into account. The size of the calculation cannot be permitted to exceed a certain voltage, the machine unit, which is governed by the type of apparatus and is generally $\pm$ 10 volts. Moreover the calculation is not accurate enough when the values are too small. All the principal and intermediate results must, therefore, remain within permitted limits. One should also establish whether the problem is to run in real time or with an altered time scale. Here, too, technology is the limiting factor.

If we think of the analogue computer as somehow having to calculate on a sheet of graph paper, then we can envisage the problem of the adjustment of amplitude and time which is involved as the task of plotting every value which arises during the calculation in a clear fashion by alterations in the scale on this graph.

3. Use

It has only recently become more common practice to describe the behaviour of a substance in the body in terms of pharmacokinetic parameters. Such information is therefore often not apparent from the literature. For example, the times needed for the blood concentration of chloramphenicol to reach a maximum after intramuscular injection and then to fall to half this value are cited in the literature. The latter time has already been shown to be different from the half-time of elimination. Further information given is the time during which the concentration remains above the necessary minimum of 10 mg/litre following a single injection of 50 mg/kg. Table 9 compares this information for children and adults, as obtained from the literature, with that for neonates. The differences are clear but the difficulty is that of predicting their importance in practical medicine.

With the help of the analogue computer, on the other hand, it is quite simple to obtain the invasion constant, the rate constant of elimination and the relative, weight-dependent volume of distribution from this information, and to show the importance of these pharmacokinetic parameters.

The lower part of Fig. 61 shows a curve which fulfils the conditions of Table 9 for children and adults. It has been obtained by continually adjusting by trial and error the potentiometers in the circuit shown in Fig. 61 which represent the coefficients k_1, k_2 and $1/V$, until the requirements were met in the ensuing curve produced on an $x - y$ plotter.

Table 9. Chloramphenicol: description of the blood concentration-time curve following an intramuscular injection of 50 mg/kg (from Walter-Heilmeyer (1975): *Antibiotika-Fibel*)

Time (hours)	Children and adults	Neonates
To reach maximum	1–2	4–5
From maximum to half maximal concentration	4–5	ca. 26
Until it falls to 10 mg/litre	10	55

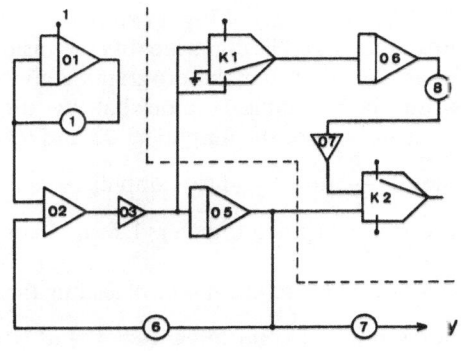

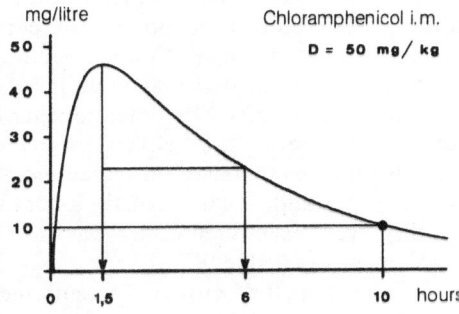

Fig. 61. *Upper figure:* trick circuit to fit the Bateman function rapidly to the conditions shown in Table 9. The programme given in Fig. 60 has been extended by the two sign-reversing amplifiers 02 and 03 (to the *left* of the *dotted line*). *K* 1 and *K* 2 are relays (comparators) which switch in when the sum of their inputs is zero. *Lower figure:* Blood concentration-time curves in children and adults after the intramuscular injection of 50 mg/kg of chloramphenicol succinate, fitted by manual adjustment of the potentiometers 1, 6 and 7. Ordinate: concentration in mg/litre Abscissa: time in hours

A digital computer can be programmed to solve the exercise with which it is presented independently and with great accuracy. In the analogue computer, the skill and judgement of the investigator decides the accuracy and time required. This disadvantage can be greatly reduced, however, by incorporating 'trick circuits'.

An example will make this clear, since it explains two important points. It shows that it is possible to express the characteristics of a model using data obtained experimentally. It also shows, however, how useful it is to regard the analogue computer as a scientific instrument or even a plaything, and thus to keep mathematics out of it.

The upper part of Fig. 61 shows a suitable circuit for the chloramphenicol problem. The digits identify the various components within the patch panel. We find that the programme given for the Bateman function has again been changed somewhat by the integrators 01 and 05. The interposition of the amplifiers 02 and 03 gives the rate of change in the blood $\frac{dB}{dt}$ directly. Two amplifiers are necessary because of the sign reversal. The potentiometers 1, 6 and 7 correspond to the coefficients k_1, k_2 and $1/V$.

The trick circuit consists of feeding the slope $\frac{dB}{dt}$ of the rising part of the curve into a second integrator (06) at whose output B can then also be measured. This information is fed in through a comparator (K 1), however, which is also governed by that rate of change. This means that the connection is broken as soon as the curve becomes horizontal, i.e. at exactly the point of reaching the maximum. From now on, the output of 06 remains constant at that maximum level.

This value is halved by potentiometer 8 and compared with B in the second comparator. K 2 delivers a signal when the amount in compartment B has fallen to half of the maximum. Since the first comparator (K 1) can deliver an additional signal, the exact time of both triggered events can be displayed exactly and, by varying k_1 and k_2, adjusted to the requirements of Table 9.

In a last step, the factor $1/V$ (potentiometer 7) can be adjusted in such a way that the curve passes through 10 mg/litre after the time indicated.

Table 10 has been obtained in this way from the values in Table 9.

The half-time of elimination of chloramphenicol is thus 6.8 times longer in neonates than in children. The half-time of invasion, however, is only approximately doubled.

When representing the conditions for repeated administration of the same dose, the effect of these differences is shown very clearly.

Figure 62 shows the blood concentrations to be expected after the 6-hourly administration of 12.5 mg/kg chloramphenicol. The curves have been calculated from an analogue computer programme which contains a circuit based on physical principles for producing a staircase-like input

Table 10. Chlorampenicol: pharmacokinetic parameters of intramuscular administration

Parameter	Children and adults	Neonates
Half-time of invasion	0.47 h	0.90 h
Half-time of elimination	3.5 h	24 h
Coefficient of distribution	0.76 litre/kg	1.05 litres/kg

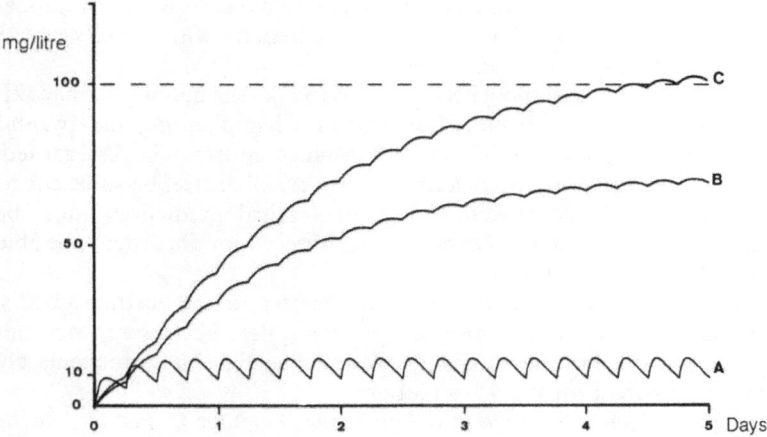

Fig. 62. Concentration-time curve for chloramphenicol succinate given intramuscularly as 4 doses a day, each of 12.5 mg/kg, in children and adults (curve A) and in neonates (curve B), based on the information in Table 10. Curve C is the concentration-time course in a hypothetical premature baby; k_{20} and the relative volume of distribution have each been reduced by 20% in comparison with the normal for mature babies. The threshold of toxicity is taken as 100 mg/litre. Ordinate: concentration (mg/litre). Abscissa: time in days

function which simulates repetitive dosage, as well as the mathematical model of the Bateman function.

Curve A represents the conditions in children and adults.

The goal of a therapeutic concentration of 10 mg/litre is achieved after the first dose of 12.5 mg/kg. The maxima and minima have already reached values after the third dose which do not change thereafter. The values for neonates are shown in curve B. The more gradual rise to considerably higher asymptotic values is largely attributable to the prolongation of the half-time of elimination, which in turn can be explained by the immaturity of the organ of elimination, the liver. The increase in the relative volume of distribution does not modify this effect to any marked extent.

Curve C is the result of a purely theoretical experiment. A hypothetical premature baby with a 20% reduction in its volume of distribution as well as impairment of its liver function by 20% because of organ immaturity receives the same weight-related dose for 5 days. The resultant blood concentration-time curve increases throughout the period of treatment and reaches the toxic concentration of 100 mg/litre on the fourth day.

The biological validity of this pharmacokinetic model is easily

113

confirmed for curves A and B by a few blood concentration studies in neonates and adults. The assumptions on which curve C is based have in the past been tragically confirmed in premature babies given chloramphenicol prophylactically, which caused severe toxicity with cardiovascular collapse, the grey syndrome.

This example shows how necessary it is to take the major pharmacokinetic parameters of a substance into account when planning therapy, and shows that the patient's individual circumstances must not be disregarded.

Mathematical procedures alone can never, of course, be sufficient to establish the validity of a model. Mathematical predictions must be correlated with the results of experimental observations in order to be able to accept or reject a model.

If a model is rejected, it is a simple matter to test further models, particularly for the user of an analogue computer. The discrepancy can often be explained in a few steps. The result of such a change immediately becomes apparent on the $x-y$ plotter.

The particular advantage of the analogue computer is therefore in the development of models. The use of this machine teaches the investigator to confine himself to circumstances of quantitative relevance and to judge the limits of the experimental system. The opportunity to simulate experiments and extrapolate them into unknown areas leads to the recognition of conditions under which biology can prove or disprove a hypothesis.

Once a pharmacokinetic model is recognised as providing an adequate answer to a problem, it should be expressed mathematically in a way convertible into a digital computer programme.

The routine evaluation of experimental results with an established mathematical model is undoubtedly the function of the digital computer on account of its greater rapidity and precision and the fact that, unlike the analogue computer, it can evaluate the statistical significance of the individual parameters.

X. Practical Application of Pharmacokinetic Procedures*

The aim of this chapter is to review some methods used in human and animal experiments in the course of the development of new drugs. Most of the examples relate to antibacterial chemotherapy, although the procedures described are not restricted to this group of drugs. The methods presented here have been confirmed in our own studies.

1. Methods of Measurement

Some brief general details are given of the different methods for constructing and evaluating concentration curves.

According to Dost (1968), pharmacokinetics is concerned with 'practical information derived from the observation of concentration-time curves of a drug and its metabolites within the compartments of the body as a whole, and in particular, the blood and urine'.

What types of method are available for this purpose?

a) Microbiological Methods

A simple in vitro test for studying the inhibitory effect of a substance directly is essential if a microbiological test method is to be used. The *advantage* of this procedure (generally the diffusion test) lies in the detection of antimicrobial activity in the substance and/or its metabolites; inactive breakdown products have no inhibitory effect. The procedure is relatively precise when suitable methods are used, and it can be related to the relevant pathogen.

The *disadvantage* of microbiological procedures is that they do not distinguish between the agent administered and those metabolites which also inhibit bacterial growth.

---
* By W.-H. Wagner, Frankfurt/M.

The *sensitivity* of the method depends on the minimal inhibitory concentration (MIC) in vitro of the test strain. This is often rather low, so that only two phases are generally detected in the concentration-time curves for blood or serum. The first phase lasts until a distribution equilibrium is established and the second phase is a straight line when plotted on semilogarithmic graph paper, i.e. it shows a simple declining exponential function. When using more sensitive methods, however, a third and perhaps even more phases have to be included, in which the half-time of elimination becomes much more prominent than in phase 2. The curve in these subsequent phases is also usually linear, however, the individual values are generally so low that they are not detectable by microbiological methods.

b) Chemical Analysis

The *advantage* of these methods is their much greater sensitivity in comparison with microbiological methods.

One *disadvantage* of chemical analysis is that new substances often require new methods of analysis which can sometimes be difficult to develop. Chemical analysis sometimes detects fractions of molecules which react as the whole molecule but possess no chemotherapeutic activity themselves; this can lead to misinterpretation.

c) Radioactively Labelled Substances

A clear *advantage* of radiolabelling is the greatly increased sensitivity in comparison with the other two methods. Such methods not only permit the measurement of concentrations in body fluids, particularly blood, plasma or serum but also provide a quite simple means of measuring excretion in the urine, stools, milk and expired air and, at the end of the experiment, of demonstrating the substance in the tissues. Thus satisfactory balance experiments become possible.

A further *advantage* is that all the metabolic products of a substance can be reliably traced even before their chemical structure is known. This greatly simplifies the detection and identification of metabolites. For this reason, measuring the 'total radioactivity' is not enough. The original substance and its metabolites must be separated from one another, for example by chromatography.

A particular, highly sensitive method is radio-immunoassay (RIA). This method makes use of the antigen-antibody reaction between the substance to be detected and an antibody specially raised against it.

Variable quantities of the substance compete with a constant amount of the same, radioactively labelled substance for a constant but limited number of antibody binding sites. After establishing an equilibrium dependent on the concentration, the antigen-antibody complex is separated from the unbound substance and the radioactivity measured in one of the two phases. The percentage of binding between radioactive molecules and antibody is then a measure of the concentration of the substance. It has been possible to raise antibodies with only slight cross-reactivity for other related substances or metabolites, so this test is very selective. Further advantages are the lack of a need for special pretreatment, so substances can be assayed directly in the biological fluid, and only very small volumes are required.

A *disadvantage* of radiochemical methods is the need to synthesise the radioactively labelled compounds. This can be costly and laborious, particularly where various positions of the molecule need to be labelled. The vital safety precautions further increase the experimental effort, and the handling of radioactive substances is closely controlled.

2. Assessment of the Results of Animal Experiments

The same rules apply to the extrapolation of the results of pharmacokinetics experiments from animals to man as are generally applicable to the results of animal experiments: no direct conclusions may be drawn from them about the behaviour of the substance in man. Similarly, the results in one animal species may differ from those in another. Thus certain sulphonamides with antibacterial activity can be short-acting in some species of animal and long-acting in others.

3. Derivation of Pharmacokinetic Parameters and Constants

a) Calculation from a Graph

Under suitable circumstances, the most important pharmacokinetic values can be found grapahically. When points are plotted semilogarithmically, the following values can be determined:

$$k_2 = \frac{\ln y_1 - \ln y_2}{t_2 - t_1} \tag{7}$$

and

$$t_{50\%} = \frac{\ln 2}{k_2} \quad (\ln 2 = 0.693) \tag{6a}$$

where y_1 and y_2 are the concentrations at times t_1 and t_2 on the declining part of the straight line.

This formula only applies to situations of pure elimination, such as follow intravenous administration. In such cases the measurements usually form a good curve. After non-intravenous, and particularly oral, administration, the curves fit less well, since the points of measurement are more scattered. The half-time of elimination ($t_{50\%}$) can be determined graphically after non-intravenous administration, however, when the resultant blood concentration-time curve is given by the Bateman function ($k_1 \gg k_2$). In these circumstances, the value of the declining portion ($t > t_{max}$) can often be treated accurately enough as a simple exponential function.

b) Programmed Procedures

For determining pharmacokinetic values and constants, programmed procedures have been introduced in the processing of measured results by large computers with fixed programmes. Unlike the use of analogue computers, these procedures do not aid the search for models; the general characteristic of the programmes is the adaptation of several e-functions to the values obtained experimentally.

We use two standard programmes. The first, based on the work of Schlender and Krüger-Thiemer (1962) but modified and extended, will determine $t_{50\%}$, k_1, k_2, r^2 and other values after intravenous administration. The second, developed by Metzler and known as Nonlin, evaluates blood concentration-time curves in situations of simultaneous invasion and elimination (Bateman function).

4. Mathematical Basis of Programming

In this section, we summarise the most important mathematical principles which underly our procedures (see also Dost, 1968).

a) Distribution of a Substance Between Several Compartments

A drug is distributed in the body according to either a single- or a multi-compartment system. Homogeneous distribution of the drug within a given compartment is assumed. The drug can be exchanged between different compartments in a way which can be expressed mathematically as a differential equation or as a system of differential equations. Let us consider a simple pharmacokinetic model in which the compartments are Cp_1, Cp_2, Cp_3 and Cp_4. Transport between these compartments is represented below by arrows between the rectangles. The values k_{ij} are rate constants.

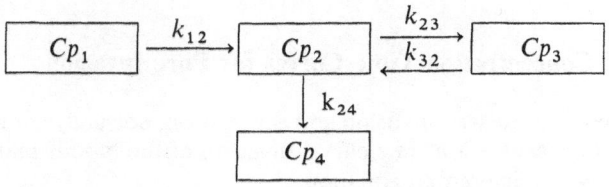

If we denote the drug concentration in a compartment at any given time as y, i.e. y_1, y_2, y_3, y_4, then the above model, which is of course one of very many possible variants, can be associated with the following series of linear differential equations:

$$\frac{dy_1}{dt} = -k_{12}y_1$$

$$\frac{dy_2}{dt} = +k_{12}y_1 - k_{23}y_2 + k_{32}y_3 - k_{224}y_2$$

$$\frac{dy_3}{dt} = \qquad\qquad +k_{23}y_2 - k_{32}y_3$$

$$\frac{dy_4}{dt} = \qquad\qquad\qquad\qquad\qquad +k_{24}y_2$$

Fig. 63. Curves of possible solutions

Assuming that the rate constants of the system are known, the series of equations can then be solved and possibly plotted out with the aid of an analogue computer and an x–y plotter.

Curves of the solutions of the equations can be plotted to give the concentration-time course in each compartment, according to the various k-values. Possible individual concentration-time curves are shown in Fig. 63.

b) Blood Concentration-Time Curves for Pure Invasion

Two different processes, invasion and elimination, normally contribute to the blood concentration-time curve. Invasion of the bloodstream by the drug obeys the differential equation:

$$\frac{dy}{dt} = k_1(y_0 - y) \tag{86}$$

$\frac{dy}{dt}$ is the rate at which the blood concentration increases and k_1 is the invasion constant. Integration after separation of the variables gives:

$$y = y_0(1 - e^{-k_1 t}) \tag{38}$$

This equation gives the *concentration-time course for pure invasion*. The blood concentration tends asymptotically towards the value of y_0. Figure 64 (left-hand graph) shows invasion curves for various values of k_1. Since these curves are sometimes required as straight lines, we give below the procedure according to which the ordinate must be subdivided to make these curves linear over the range required.

$$y = y_0(1 - e^{-k_1 t})$$

$$y - y_0 = -y_0 \cdot e^{-k_1 t}$$

$$\frac{y - y_0}{y_0} = -e^{-k_1 t} \tag{87}$$

$$\ln \frac{y_0 - y}{y_0} = -k_1 t$$

$$\ln \frac{y_0}{y_0 - y} = k_1 t$$

Subdivision of the ordinates in this way gives straight lines with a slope of k_1 (Fig. 64, right-hand graph).

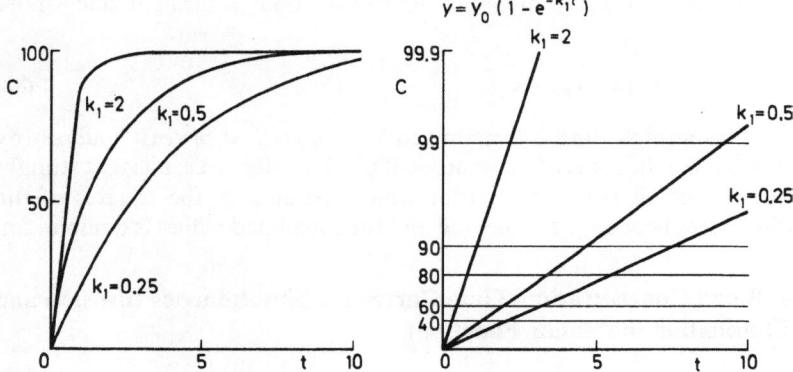

Fig. 64. Invasion

c) Blood Concentration-Time Curves for Pure Elimination

Blood concentration-time curves following the intravenous administration of a drug are associated with the following differential equation:

$$\frac{dy}{dt} = -k_2 y \tag{4}$$

This is a process of pure elimination and k_2 is the rate constant of elimination. This differential equation can also be solved by the method of separation of variables to yield:

$$y = y_0 \cdot e^{-k_2 t} \tag{5}$$

Where the process is one of elimination only, the half-time ($t_{50\%}$) of elimination can be calculated. This is the time taken for the blood concentration to fall to one-half. We obtain:

$$\frac{\ln 2}{k_2} = t_{50\%} \tag{6a}$$

A frequent practical problem is the determination of y_0 and k_2 from blood concentrations which have been measured at different times. The situation is as follows:

n pairs of measurements are given $(t_1, y_1); (t_2, y_2); \ldots (t_n, y_n)$. Naturally, these points do not all lie on an exponential curve, since the values $y_1, y_2, \ldots y_n$ are subject to experimental error. Substitution with $\ln y_i$ in place of y_i

gives rise to a series of points scattered about a straight line whose equation is:

$$\ln y = \ln y_0 - k_2 t \tag{88}$$

This straight line is determined by the *method of least squares* (by minimizing the sums of the squares of the deviations), i.e. it is that straight line out of all possible lines for which the sum of the squares of the differences between the observed and the calculated values is a minimum.

d) Blood Concentration-Time Curves for Simultaneous Invasion and Elimination (Bateman Function)

The following model applies to simultaneous invasion and elimination such as follows *non-intravenous* administration:

$$\boxed{X} \xrightarrow{k_1} \boxed{Y} \xrightarrow{k_2}$$

X is the compartment from which invasion into the bloodstream occurs and Y represents the compartment 'blood'.

The following series of differential equations can be drawn up:

$$\frac{dX}{dt} = -k_1 X \tag{35}$$

$$\frac{dY}{dt} = +k_1 X - k_2 \cdot Y \tag{39}$$

From the first equation,

$$X = X_0 \cdot e^{-k_1 t},$$

i.e. there is an exponential fall in compartment X.

Using this result, the second equation takes the form:

$$\frac{dY}{dt} = k_1 \cdot X_0 \cdot e^{-k_1 t} - k_2 \cdot Y$$

We can solve this differential equation by the method of integrating factors:

$$\frac{dY}{dt} + k_2 Y = k_1 X_0 e^{-k_1 t \cdot} \mid e^{k_2 t}$$

$$\frac{dY}{dt} \cdot e^{k_2 t} + k_2 \cdot Y e^{k_2 t} = k_1 X_0 e^{(k_2 - k_1)t}$$

$$\frac{d(Y \cdot e^{k_2 t})}{dt} = k_1 X_0 \cdot e^{(k_2 - k_1)t}$$

$$Y \cdot e^{k_2 t} = k_1 X_0 \cdot \int_0^t e^{(k_2 - k_1)t}$$

$$Y \cdot e^{k_2 t} = \frac{k_1 X_0}{k_2 - k_1}(e^{(k_2 - k_1)t} - 1)$$

$$Y = \frac{k_1 X_0}{k_2 - k_1}(e^{-k_1 t} - e^{-k_2 t})$$

from which we can also write, using the original terms:

$$y = \frac{k_1 \cdot y_0}{k_1 - k_2}(e^{-k_2 t} - e^{-k_1 t}) \tag{40}$$

This function has become known in pharmacokinetics as the Bateman function.

As in the case of pure elimination metioned above, the requirement in practice is that of constructing a theoretical curve through measured points such that the sum of the square of the deviations is a minimum (Fig. 65).

Given the pairs of measured values $(t_1, y_1); (t_2, y_2); \ldots; (t_n, y_n)$, the indices y_0, k_1 and k_2 are required, such that

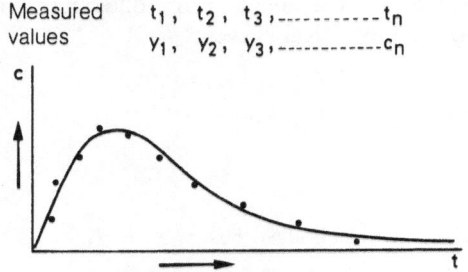

Fig. 65. The problem of adjustment

Measured values: $t_1, t_2, t_3, \ldots t_n$; $y_1, y_2, y_3, \ldots c_n$

The parameters y_0, k_1 and k_2 of the Bateman function must be so determined that

$$Q = \sum_i \left[y_i - \frac{k_1 y_0}{k_1 - k_2}(e^{-k_2 t_i} - e^{-k_1 t_i}) \right]^2 \to \min$$

$$Q = Q(y_0, k_1, k_2) = \sum \left[y_i - \frac{y_0 k_1}{k_1 - k_2} (e^{-k_2 t_i} - e^{k_1 t_i}) \right]^2 \to \text{Min.} \quad (89)$$

This problem is not so easy to solve as that of the linear function, since the factors required are not completely rational functions, but rather exponents in a sum of exponential functions.

The values of y_0, k_1 and k_2 can be calculated from the pairs of measured values in an experiment by using the Gauss-Newton iteration procedure.

Let us state the problem:

From the paired data $(t_i; y_i)$ a function must be found which has the following form:

$$y = F(y_0, k_1, k_2, t) = \frac{k_1 \cdot y_0}{k_1 - k_2} (e^{-k_2 t} - e^{-k_1 t}) \quad (90)$$

The following abbreviations may be introduced:

$F(y_0, k_1, k_2, t_i) = F_i(y_0, k_1, k_2)$, i.e. as an indication that we are dealing with the value of the function at time t_i, we introduce an index i for the functional symbol F. In the ideal situation, therefore,

$$\begin{aligned} F_1(y_0, k_1, k_2) &= y_1 \\ F_2(y_0, k_1, k_2) &= y_2 \\ &\vdots \\ F_n(y_0, k_1, k_2) &= y_n, \end{aligned} \quad (91)$$

i.e. the function $F(y_0, k_1, k_2, t)$ passes through all the measured points. Since we are now dealing with blood concentrations whose measurement is subject to experimental error, differences v_i are found between the actual and the theoretical curves:

$$\begin{aligned} F_1(y_0, k_1, k_2) - y_1 &= v_1 \\ F_2(y_0, k_1, k_2) - y_2 &= v_2 \\ &\vdots \\ F_n(y_0, k_1, k_2) - y_n &= v_n \end{aligned} \quad (92)$$

Our claim is that:

$$\sum_{i=1}^{n} v_i^2 \to \text{Min.} \quad (93)$$

The parameters y_0, k_1 and k_2 are now determined by assuming primary estimates for them which can possibly be obtained from a graph. Let us designate these approximations as

$$y_0^{(0)}, k_1^{(0)}, k_2^{(0)}$$

Starting from these approximations, correcting factors $\Delta y_0, \Delta k_1, \Delta k_2$ are calculated which, when added to the zeroeth approximations, yield improved (secondary) estimates.

$$\begin{aligned} y_0^{(1)} &= y_0^{(0)} + \Delta y_0 \\ k_1^{(1)} &= k_1^{(0)} + \Delta k_1 \\ k_2^{(1)} &= k_2^{(0)} + \Delta k_2 \end{aligned} \qquad (94)$$

The new approximations are now used in place of the old values. How are the correcting factors $\Delta y_0, \Delta k_1, \Delta k_2$ calculated? One transforms the function into a Taylor series using only the first-order derivatives

$$F_i(y_0, k_1, k_2) = F_i(y_0^{(0)}, k_1^{(0)}, k_2^{(0)}) + \left(\frac{\partial F_i}{\partial y_0}\right)_0 \cdot \Delta y_0 + \left(\frac{\partial F_i}{\partial k_1}\right)_0 \cdot \Delta k_1 + \left(\frac{\partial F_i}{\partial k_2}\right)_0 \cdot \Delta k_2$$

The figure 0 in the partial derivations shows that the derivations should be formed for the primary estimates.

If we substitute v_i in the equation, then

$$F_1(y_0, k_1, k_2) - y_1 = F_1(y_0^{(0)}, k_1^{(0)}, k_2^{(0)}) + \left(\frac{\partial F_1}{\partial y_0}\right)_0 \Delta y_0$$
$$+ \left(\frac{\partial F_1}{\partial k_1}\right)_0 \Delta k_1 + \left(\frac{\partial F_1}{\partial k_2}\right)_0 \Delta k_2 - y_1 \qquad (95)$$

$$F_2(y_0, k_1, k_2) - y_2 = F_2(y_0^{(0)}, k_1^{(0)}, k_2^{(0)}) + \left(\frac{\partial F_2}{\partial y_0}\right)_0 \Delta y_0$$
$$+ \left(\frac{\partial F_2}{\partial k_1}\right)_0 \Delta k_1 + \left(\frac{\partial F_2}{\partial k_2}\right)_0 \Delta k_2 - y_2$$

$$\vdots$$

$$F_n(y_0, k_1, k_2) - y_n = F_n(y_0^{(0)}, k_1^{(0)}, k_2^{(0)}) + \left(\frac{\partial F_n}{\partial y_0}\right)_0 \Delta y_0$$
$$+ \left(\frac{\partial F_n}{\partial k_1}\right)_0 \Delta k_1 + \left(\frac{\partial F_n}{\partial k_2}\right)_0 \Delta k_2 - y_n$$

This system of linear equations has more equations than unknowns. The unknown values Δy_0, Δk_1 and Δk_2 can be found by using the following series of normal equations:

$$\Delta y_0 \cdot \sum_{i=1}^{n} \left(\frac{\partial F_i}{\partial y_0}\right)\left(\frac{\partial F_i}{\partial y_0}\right) + \Delta k_1 \cdot \sum_{i=1}^{n} \left(\frac{\partial F_i}{\partial y_0}\right)\left(\frac{\partial F_i}{\partial k_1}\right) +$$

$$+ \Delta k_2 \cdot \sum_{i=1}^{n} \left(\frac{\partial F_i}{\partial y_0}\right)\left(\frac{\partial F_i}{\partial k_2}\right) = \sum_{i=1}^{n} \left(\frac{\partial F_i}{\partial y_0}\right) \cdot l_i$$

$$\Delta y_0 \cdot \sum_{i=1}^{n} \left(\frac{\partial F_i}{\partial y_0}\right) \cdot \left(\frac{\partial F_i}{\partial k_1}\right) + \Delta k_1 \cdot \sum_{i=1}^{n} \cdot \left(\frac{\partial F_i}{\partial k_1}\right) \cdot \left(\frac{\partial F_i}{\partial k_1}\right) + \qquad (96)$$

$$+ \Delta k_2 \cdot \sum_{i=1}^{n} \left(\frac{\partial F_i}{\partial k_1}\right) \cdot \left(\frac{\partial F_i}{\partial k_2}\right) = \sum_{i=1}^{n} \left(\frac{\partial F_i}{\partial k_1}\right) \cdot l_i$$

$$\Delta y_0 \cdot \sum_{i=1}^{n} \left(\frac{\partial F_1}{\partial y_0}\right) \cdot \left(\frac{\partial F_i}{\partial k_2}\right) + \Delta k_1 \cdot \sum_{i=1}^{n} \cdot \left(\frac{\partial F_i}{\partial k_1}\right) \cdot \left(\frac{\partial F_i}{\partial k_2}\right) +$$

$$+ \Delta k_2 \cdot \sum_{i=1}^{n} \left(\frac{\partial F_i}{\partial k_2}\right) \cdot \left(\frac{\partial F_i}{\partial k_2}\right) = \sum_{i=1}^{n} \left(\frac{\partial F_1}{\partial k_2}\right) \cdot l_i$$

Here, l_i stands for the quantity $F_i(y_0^{(0)}, k_1^{(0)}, k_2^{(0)}) - y_i$. From this system of normal equations, the quantities Δy_0, Δk_1 and Δk_2 can be determined.

A computer programme also tests in the calculation whether these corrections are worthwhile in the context of the precision which we require. This is decided by a test, where the following should apply:

$$\left|\frac{\Delta y_0}{y_0}\right| + \left|\frac{\Delta k_1}{k_1}\right| + \left|\frac{\Delta k_2}{k_2}\right| < \varepsilon, \qquad (97)$$

where ε is a limit of precision given in advance by the programme user.

e) Accumulation, Limiting Curve

If the three parameters y_0, k_1 and k_2 have been determined in the manner just described, one can calculate the blood concentration which should be substituted when giving the same dose repeatedly at constant time intervals, τ. The resultant curve is called a cumulation curve if τ is small in comparison with $t_{50\%}$.

f) Dosage Scheme

Let us assume the Bateman function:

$$y(t) = \frac{y_0 k_1}{k_1 - k_2} (e^{-k_2 t} - e^{-k_1 t}) \tag{40}$$

This would be the blood concentration curve obtained after nonintravenous administration of the initial dose D^*.

After time τ has elapsed, the following value is obtained:

$$y(\tau) = \frac{y_0 k_1}{k_1 - k_2} (e^{-k_2 \tau} - e^{-k_1 \tau})$$

Figure 66 explains what is to be understood by the maintenance dose, D.

D is the dose which should be given after times $\tau, 2\tau, 3\tau \ldots$ so that the blood concentration at the end of each dose-interval is always the same: $y(\tau)$.

5. Examples of Calculations

A few examples will be given to clarify the ways in which the calculation procedures outlined under Sections 3.a. and 3.b. of this chapter can be used. Simple blood concentration-time curves are used for this purpose; the analysis of complex concentration curves and the extension to other compartments is deliberately avoided.

Example 1 shows how most values of pharmacokinetic interest can be read off or calculated directly from the graph when the individual points have been measured accurately enough. The serum concentration-time

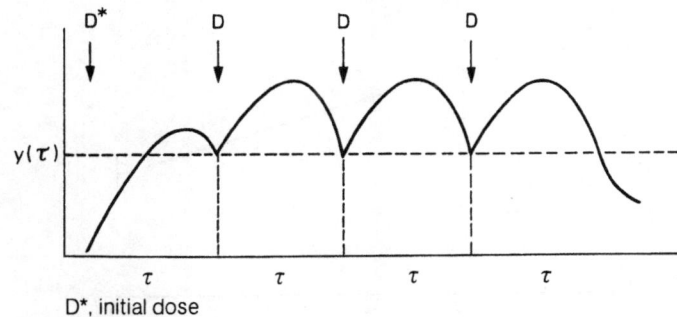

D*, initial dose
D, maintenance dose

Fig. 66. Blood concentration-time curves for multiple dosing

curves given here were obtained following the intravenous administration of pyrrolidinomethyltetracycline. These are curves of mean values; five male and five female volunteers were studied for these experiments (Figs. 67–69) (Dimmling and Wagner, 1965).

Thus the values for the curve and half-time of elimination can be determined easily from the mean curves for five male and five female volunteers (Fig. 67) by using the formulae given under Section 3.a. of this chapter:

$$k_2 = 0.087 \text{ h}^{-1}$$
$$t_{50\%} = 7.77 \text{ h}$$

As already mentioned, the curves after intravenous administration are better defined because there are no individual variations in the rate of absorption such as are found after non-intravenous administration.

The analysis of the scatter found in the curves of mean concentration is of interest; Figs. 67–69 show three serum concentration curves from the experiment mentioned together with the standard errors of the means.

Table 11 shows the coefficients of variation for various times:

$$V = \frac{s}{x} \cdot 100$$

In *example 2*, a programmed procedure was used. The substance was given as a single dose of 150 mg/kg i.v.; the calculation is based on a *one-compartment model*. The values lying on the log-linear declining part of the

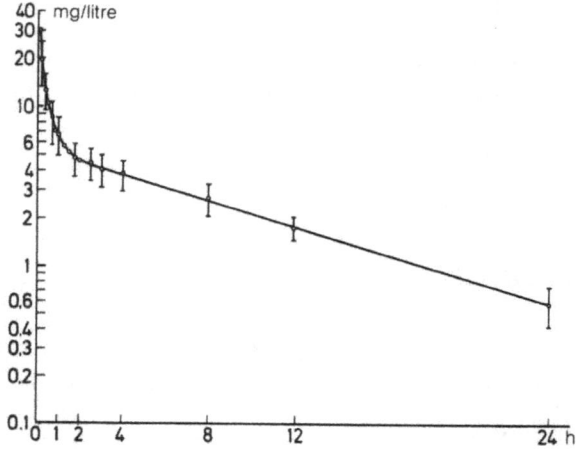

Fig. 67. Comparative blood concentration-time curves after a single intravenous dose of 275 mg pyrrolidinomethyltetracycline. Mean values for five male and five female subjects

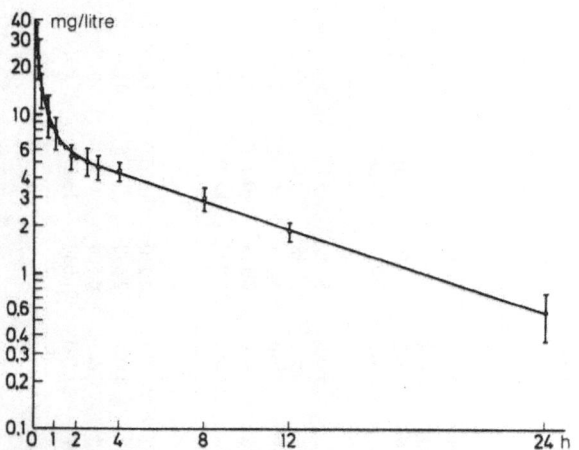

Fig. 68. Comparative blood concentration-time curves after a single intravenous dose of 275 mg pyrrolidinomethyltetracycline. Mean value for five female volunteers

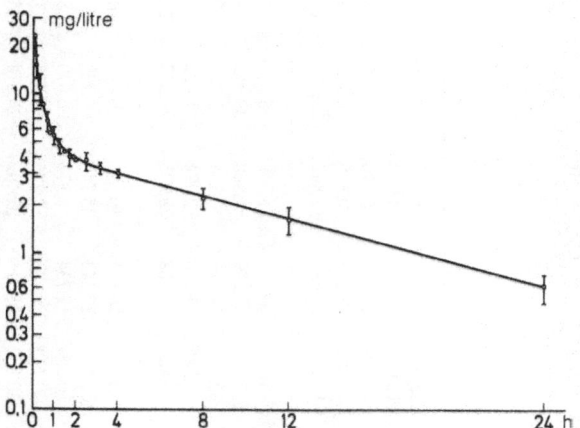

Fig. 69. Comparative blood concentration-time curve after a single intravenous dose of 175 mg pyrrolidinomethyltetracycline. Mean value for five male volunteers

curve are used for the calculation. Figure 70 shows the curve again and Table 12 gives the print-out of the pharmacokinetic values and constants as determined by an electronic digital computer.

Table 11. Comparative studies of blood concentrations after a single intravenous dose of 275 mg pyrrolidinomethyltetracycline

Sex		5'	20'	40'	60'	90'	120'	180'	8 h	12 h	24 h
	No.	5	5	5	5	5	5	5	4	4	4
	Total[a]	115.946	54.764	34.079	27.690	21.938	19.398	17.361	9.042	6.610	2.511
	$\bar{x}$[a]	23.189	10.953	6.816	5.538	4.388	3.880	3.472	2.260	1.652	0.628
	Standard error[a]	2.582	2.259	0.875	0.737	0.453	0.416	0.262	0.318	0.319	0.114
	Coefficient of variation[b]	11.134	20.629	12.842	13.315	10.324	10.711	7.542	14.052	19.288	18.166
	No.	5	5	5	5	5	5	5	5	5	5
	Total[a]	187.595	72.579	51.668	39.012	31.241	26.979	23.552	15.168	9.461	2.922
	$\bar{x}$	37.519	14.516	10.334	7.802	6.248	5.395	4.710	3.034	1.892	0.584
	Standard error	7.286	3.158	2.994	1.822	1.313	0.930	0.814	0.483	0.247	0.212
	Coefficient of variation	19.420	21.758	28.975	23.357	21.008	17.242	17.282	15.907	13.040	36.236
	No.	10	10	10	10	10	10	10	9	9	9
	Total	303.541	127.343	85.747	66.702	53.179	46.372	40.913	24.210	16.071	5.433
	$\bar{x}$	30.354	12.734	8.575	6.670	5.318	4.637	4.091	2.690	1.786	0.604
	Standard error	9.143	3.198	2.786	1.773	1.349	1.048	0.867	0.566	0.291	0.167
	Coefficient of variation	30.122	25.115	32.492	26.574	25.359	22.607	21.180	21.039	16.279	27.631

[a] Results in mg/litre
[b] Results in %

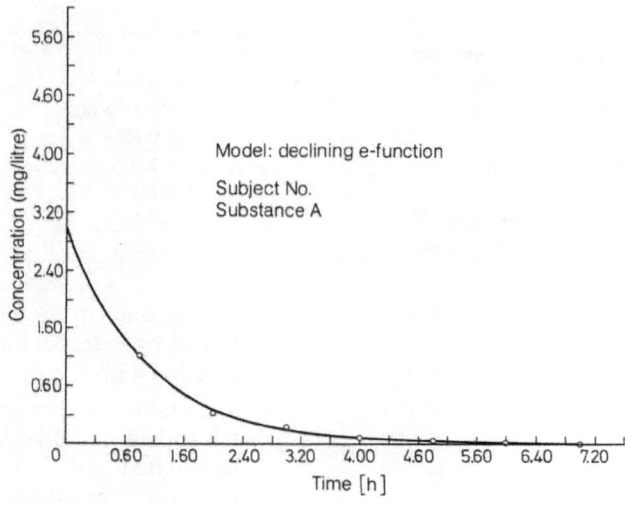

Fig. 70. Graph of the curve obtained from example 2

Table 12. Print-out of the results of example 2 (Nonlin). See text for details

Kinetic Results

Model used: Declining e-function
Date of experiment: 23. 6. 76   Species: Man
Experiment number: 527   Body weight: 70.00 kg
Subject number: 14   Material studied: serum
Drug: Substance a
Dose: 150.00 mg/kg
Total dose: 10500.00 mg
Mode of administration: i.v.
Remarks: 0

Time h	Measured conc. (mg/litre)	Calculated conc. (mg/litre)	Weight
1.000	1.221	1.210	1.000
2.000	0.432	0.483	1.000
3.000	0.242	0.193	1.000
4.000	0.090	0.077	1.000
5.000	0.051	0.031	1.000
6.000	0.019	0.012	1.000
7.000	0.010	0.005	1.000

Table 12 (cont.)

Pharmacokinetic Constants		
Initial concentration	3.026	µg/ml
Elimination constant	0.917e 00	litres/h
corresponding $t_{50\%}$	0.756	h
Area under the curve	3.300	µg/h/ml
r squared	0.997	
Volume of distribution	3469.567	litre
Coefficient of distribution	49.565	litres/kg

Definitions:

Initial concentration (y_0): Initial concentration at time t_0 obtained by extrapolation $t_0 = 0$

Elimination constant (k_2): A value with the dimension h^{-1}

Half-time of elimination ($t_{50\%}$): Time taken for the concentration to fall to half its initial value

Area under the curve: Calculated with the aid of the turnover equation of Dost; dimension:
$$\frac{\mu g \cdot h}{ml}$$

$$r^2 = 1 - \frac{\sum [y_{obs}(t_i) - F(t_i)]^2}{\sum [\bar{y}_{obs} - y_{obs}(t_i)]^2}$$

r^2 is the measure of the degree to which the calculated curve $F(t)$ fits the measured points $(t, y_{obs}(t_i))$, i.e. it is a measure of the exactness with which it is possible to express the scatter of points obtained experimentally in the form of a curve.

The values in the column 'calculated conc. (mg/litre)' in the print-out in Table 12 are those which lie on the curve $F(t_i)$ calculated by the method of least squares; the first value is extrapolated.

Volume of distribution: According to the single-compartment model assumed, the total dose D is distributed immediately and uniformly into this first compartment of volume V so that the concentration there is y_0.
$y_0 = D/V$
and
$V = D/y_0$. Dimension: litre

Coefficient of distribution: Volume of distribution in relation to the body weight.
$\Delta = V/G$ Dimension: litres/kg

In *example 3*, 30 mg/kg substance A is given intramuscularly. The model has two compartments and the Bateman function is used to calculate the pharmacokinetics.

Table 13. Print-out of the results of example 3 (Nonlin): see text for details

Kinetic Results

Model used: Bateman function
Date of experiment: 10. 11. 69   Species: Rabbit
Experiment number: 222   Body weight: 1.00 kg
Subject number: 0   Material studied: serum
Drug: Substance a
Dose: 30.00 mg/kg
Total dose: 30.00 mg
Mode of
administration: i.m.
Remarks: 0

Time h	Measured conc. (mg/litre)	Calculated conc. (mg/litre)	Weight
0.010	1.400	0.064	1.000
0.250	2.100	1.394	1.000
0.500	2.780	2.424	1.000
1.000	4.200	3.734	1.000
2.000	4.200	4.751	1.000
3.500	4.900	4.879	1.000
7.000	3.900	4.243	1.000
12.000	3.350	3.375	1.000
16.000	2.950	2.809	1.000
20.000	2.500	2.338	1.000
24.000	2.100	1.946	1.000

Pharmacokinetic Constants

theoretical initial concentration	5.619	µg/ml
Invasion constant:	1.148	litres/h
corresponding $t_{50\%}$	0.604	h
Elimination constant:	0.459e-01	litres/h
corresponding $t_{50\%}$	15.110	h
Time lag in invasion	0.000	h
Real half-time	18.921	h
Position of peak for single dose		
Time	2.921	h
Height	4.914	µg/ml
Area under the curve	122.491	µg/h/ml
r squared	0.974	

Definitions from the print-out (Table 13) are:

Theoretical initial concentration (y_0):	Calculated starting concentration. Dimension: mg/litre
Invasion constant (k_1):	Rate constant for the transfer from the first to the second compartment. Dimension: h^{-1}
Elimination constant (k_2):	Rate constant for elimination from the second compartment. Dimension: h^{-1}
Delay in invasion t_0:	Time lag between the administration into the first compartment and invasion from the first to the second compartments. Dimension: h
Real half-time:	Time after which the concentration $y(t)$ has fallen to half its maximum value, after a single dose. Dimension: h
Position of peak for single dose:	Time of the maximum value for the Bateman function is: $$t_{max} = \frac{\ln k_1 - \ln k_2}{k_1 - k_2} + t_0$$ Its peak value is: $$y_{max} = y_0 \left[\frac{k_1}{k_2} \right]^{\frac{k_2}{k_2 - k_1}}$$
Area under the curve (AUC):	Dimension: h/mg/litre
r^2	See above

In cases of repeated administration of the same dose it is important to determine the ratio of the initial dose to the maintenance dose. The object is to calculate a dosage regimen for which the concentration does not fall below minimal values. Thus the limiting minimal value depends on the size of the initial dose and the length of the dose-interval. The calculated dose ratio guarantees a periodic curve in which the same minimal concentration is always achieved at the end of the dose-interval. The experimenter must decide where to set y_{min}, taking such things as the minimal inhibitory concentration of the chemotherapeutic agent in vitro into account. The size of the initial dose and the length of the dose-interval are worked out accordingly.

When the same dose D is given often enough at a constant dose interval τ, a concentration y_{min} is found at the end of every dose-interval. This concentration is called the minimal cumulative concentration:

$$y_{min} = \frac{y_0 \cdot k_1}{k_1 - k_2} \cdot \left[\frac{1}{1 - e^{-k_2 \tau}} - \frac{1}{1 - e^{-k_1 \tau}} \right] \qquad (98)$$

The concentration curve also repeats itself within each subsequent dose-interval, as described by the following equation:

$$y_{max} = \frac{y_0 \cdot k_1}{k_1 - k_2} \cdot \left[\frac{e^{-k_2 t'_{max}}}{1 - e^{-k_1 \tau}} - \frac{e^{-k_1 t'_{max}}}{1 - e^{-k_1 \tau}} \right] \qquad (99)$$

where t'_{max} is the time taken during the dose-interval to reach the maximum concentration. This is the maximal cumulative concentration.

With repeated dosage, therefore, a periodicity is achieved after a certain time. The repeated dose D is called the maintenance dose. If the equations for y_{min} and y_{max} are combined, it becomes clear that the ratio $y_{min} : y_{max}$ is independent of the theoretical initial concentration y_0. If k_1 and k_2 are known as well as y_{min} and y_{max}, the ratio $y_{min} : y_{max}$ can be determined for the appropriate dose-interval τ.

Once these are known, the related theoretical initial concentration y_0 can be determined approximately from the equation for y_{min}. Since the volume of distribution V is known and predetermined as a constant, the maintenance dose can be calculated from

$$D = y_0 \cdot V$$

The periodic process mentioned above can be described as follows. Known values of y_{min}, y_{max} and the volume of distribution V are associated with a maintenance dose D and a dose-interval τ. If a dose D is given at concentration y_{min}, the concentration increases to y_{max} and then falls back again to y_{min} after time τ.

Another illustration (non-intravenous administration) shows again the relationship between initial and maintenance doses. Three different curves are plotted in Fig. 71. It is assumed that the same substance is given by the same route but in different doses. An attempt is made not to fall below a particular value of y_{min}. Since the same substance is always involved, the values for k_1 and k_2 are the same in every case. The desired effect can be achieved by varying the length of the dose-interval. If this is too short, smaller doses can be used both initially and for maintenance. If the dose-interval is prolonged, higher doses should be given which produce higher peaks. Each case must be considered separately so as not to exceed the tolerable maximum whilst still ensuring that the dosage regimen is practicable.

Our last example (4) shows the accumulation of a chemotherapeutic agent, in this case streptomycin sulphate, when $\tau < t_{50\%}$ (Fig. 72).

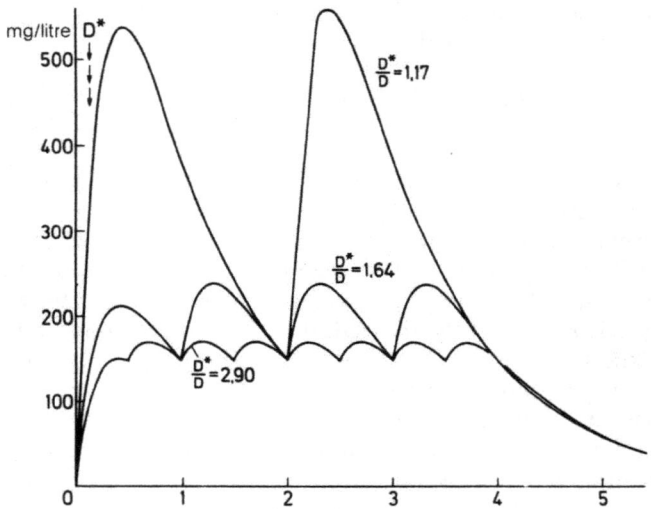

Fig. 71. Curves of repeated dosage and different dose intervals

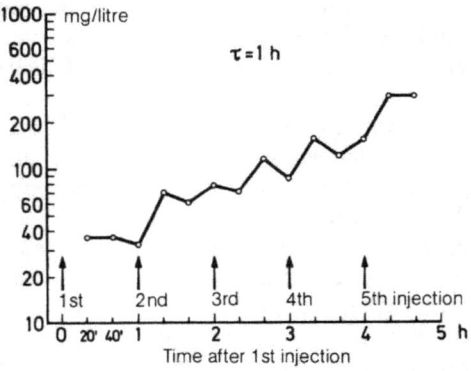

Fig. 72. Accumulation of streptomycin sulphate after five doses of 10 mg/kg i. m. in the rabbit

Further Reading

Monographs

Dengler, H. J. (ed.): Pharmacological and clinical significance of Pharmacokinetics. Stuttgart, New York: Schattauer 1970
Dost, F. H.: Der Blutspiegel. Leipzig: VEB Thieme 1953
Dost, F. H.: Grundlagen der Pharmakokinetik. Stuttgart: Thieme 1968
Gilette, J. R., Mitchell, J. R.: Concepts in Biochemical Pharmacology Part 3. Berlin, Heidelberg, New York: Springer 1975
Raspe, G. (ed.): Schering workshop on Pharmacokinetics, Advances in the Biosciences 5. Braunschweig: Pergamon Press-Vieweg 1970
Ritschel, W. A.: Handbook of Basic Pharmacokinetics. Hamilton: Drug Intelligence Publications 1976
Röpke, H., Riemann J.: Analogcomputer in Chemie und Biologie. Berlin, Heidelberg, New York: Springer 1969
Stacy, R. W., Waxman B. (ed.): Computers in biomedical research. New York, London: Academic Press 1965
Wagner, J. G.: Biopharmaceutics and relevant pharmacokinetics. 1st. ed. Hamilton: Drug Intelligence Publications 1971
Walter, A. M., Heilmeyer, L. Antibiotikafibel 4. Aufl. Stuttgart Thieme 1975

Journals

European Journal of Clinical Pharmacology. Berlin, Heidelberg, New York: Springer
International Journal of Clinical Pharmacology, Therapy and Toxicology. München, Berlin, Wien: Urban & Schwarzenberg
Journal of Pharmacokinetics and Biopharmaceutics. New York, London: Plenum-Press

Articles

Dimmling, Th., Wagner, W. H.: Konzentrationen von Tetracyclinen im Serum nach oraler und intravenöser Gabe. Arzneim. Forsch. **15**, 1288 (1965)
Dost, F. H.: Transfer und Transit als pharmakokinetische Mengenbeziehungen in einem Multikompartiment-Modell. Dtsch. med. Wochenschr. **94**, 1713 (1970)
Dost, F. H.: Eine pharmakokinetische Funktion für die Galenik. Arzneim. Forsch. **21**, 712 (1971)
Gibaldi, M., Nagashima, R., Levy, G.: Relationship between drug concentration in plasma or serum and amount of drug in the body. J. Pharm. Sci. **58**, 193–197 (1969)
Kellner, H.-M., Christ, O., Rupp, W., Heptner, W.: Resorption, Verteilung und Ausscheidung nach Gabe von ^{14}C-markiertem HB 419 an Kaninchen, Ratten und Hunden. Arzneim. Forsch. **19**, 1388 (1969)
Krüger-Thiemer, E.: Theorie der Wirkung bakteriostatischer Chemotherapeutica. Jber. Borstel **5**, 316 (1961)

Krüger-Thiemer, E., Eriksen, S. P. Mathematical model of sustained release preparations and its analysis. J. Pharm. Sci. **55**:1249 (1966)

Kübler, W.: Pharmakokinetische Methoden zur Ermittlung der enteralen Resorption. Z. Kinderheil. **108**, 187–196 (1970)

Kübler, W., Gehler, J.: Zur Kinetik der enteralen Ascorbinsäure-Resorption. Ein Beitrag zur Berechnung nicht dosisproportionierter Resorptionsvorgänge. Int. Z. Vitaminforsch. **40**, 442–453 (1970)

Lineweaver, H., Burk, D.: The determination of enzyme dissociation constants. J. Am. Chem. Soc. **56**, 658–666 (1934)

Metzler, C. M. Nonlin: A computer program for parameter estimation in nonlinear situations. Kalamazoo, Mich. The Upjohn Co. techn. rep. 7292/69/7292/005 (1969)

Riegelmann, S., Loo, J. C. K., Rowland, M.: Shortcomings in pharmacokinetic analysis by conceiving the body to exhibit properties of a single compartment. J. Pharm. Sci. **57**, 117–123 (1968)

Schlender, B., Krüger-Thiemer, E.: Die Lösung chemotherapeutischer Probleme durch programmgesteuerte Ziffernrechenautomaten. Arzneim. Forsch. **12**, 992 (1962)

Teorell, T.: Kinetics of distribution of substances administered to the body. Arch. Int. Pharmacodyn. Ther. **57**, 206 and 226 (1937)

Wagner, W.-H., Chou, J. T. Y., Ilberg, Ch. v., Ritter, R., Vosteen K. H.: Untersuchungen zur Pharmakokinetik von Streptomycin. Arzneim. Forsch. **21**, 2006–2016 (1971)

Wagner, J. G., Northam, J. I.: Estimation of distribution and half-life of a compound after rapid intravenous injection. J. Pharm. Sci. **56**, 529–531 (1967)

Subject Index

Absorption, dose-dependent 84
–, dose-proportional 78
–, gastrointestinal 68
–, site of 80
Absorption constant 38
Absorptive capacity 84, 87
Accumulation 126
Acetylaminophenol 92
Acid 95
Acid-base balance 94
Administration, repeated 63
Adsorbants 101
Alkaloids 95
Amplifier 106
Analogue computer programm 108
Analogue computers 104
Analogy 39
Antibacterial chemotherapy 115
Anticoagulant therapy 95
Antipyrine 3
Areas 57
–, corresponding 43, 72
–, corresponding fractional 49
–, determination of 46
–, fractional 50
–, rule of corresponding 43
Ascites 103
Ascorbic acid
Availments 52
Azorubin 92

Barbiturates 39, 39, 68, 68, 95
Bases 95, 95
Bateman function 39, 42, 68, 108, 118, 122
– –, distortion of 71
Benzathine penicillin 42
Bile 9
Bilirubin 25, 30, 92, 95
Biological half-life 57

Biopharmaceutics 37
Body water 3
Briggsian logarithms 14
Bromsulphalein 7, 15, 83, 92, 93, 99

C; 55
Capacitors 106
Caronamide 101
Cephalosporins 7
Cerebrospinal fluid (CSF) 5
Chelating agents 101
Chephaloridine 92
Chloramphenicol 110, 113
Chromium-EDTA 61
Circadian rhythm 95
Clearance 16, 57
–, creatinine 24, 92
–, endogenous 30
–, total 16
Clearance depression 57, 101
Compartment 36
Compartment, central 36
Compartments, transcellular 3
Computer 104
Concentration, initial 12
– y^*, basal 26
Constant, elimination 57
Constants, hybrid 54
Contrast media 92
Creatinine 92
Cumulative residue 65
Curve-peeling 56

Degree of Accumulation 65
Dehydration 102
Depot preparation 37
Dicoumarol 95
Digital computers 104
Distribution 53
–, central volume of 59

139

Distribution, coefficient of 3, 132
–, total volume of 59
–, volume of 1, 58, 102, 132
Dosage scheme 127
Dose, loading 33
–, priming 33
Dose-interval, relative 65
Dost's Principle 43, 43
Doxycycline 8, 101
Duration of accumulation 63

Elderly 94
Elimination 9, 121
–, half-time of 13, 32
Emptying 71
Endoplasmic reticulum 95
Enzyme induction 95
Equations, normal 126
Ethambutol 92
Ethanol 3, 19, 28
Excess 27
Extracellular fluid (ECF) 3, 5

Feathering 56
Function, multi-exponential 54
Function tests 15

Glomerular filtration 9, 92, 93
Glucoronidation 99
Glucose 25, 30
– excess 27
Glucuronidation 94
Glucuronyl transferase 94, 95
Grey syndrome 114
Half-time 13, 32, 57
Hepatocellular disease 92
Hydration 102
Hydrocephalus 103
Hydrothorax 103

Inactivators 94
Indocyanine 100
– green 15, 17, 93
Infusion, chronic intravenous 22
–, intravenous 58
–, rate of 49
Initial dose 134
Insecticides 95
Interaction 91
Intestinal segment 70
Intracellular fluid volume (ICF) 3

Inulin 15, 61, 92
Invasion 37, 120
–, completness 42, 45
Invasion constant k 38
Invasion curve 38
Invasion curves, reconstruction of 72
Iron 8, 25, 30
–, oral 51
Iron deficiency 51
Isoniazid 92
Isonicotinic acid hydrzide 94

Jaundice, haemolytic 25
–, hepatocellular 25
–, neonatal 101
–, obstructive 25

k_2 14
kel 58
Kernicterus 95, 101

Labelled substances 116
Langmuir isotherm 6
Law of mass action 6, 100
Lipoprotein 82
Logarithm 14, 14
Lymphatic transport 81

Maintenance dose 135
Mass action, law of 6, 100
Michaelis Menten 17, 85
Microconstants 54
Morphine 95
Multicompartment systems 35, 67

Neonate 93
Newborn 95
Nikethamide 95
Nitrofurantoin 92, 92, 101
Nonlin 118, 131

Para-aminobenzoic acid 92
Para-aminohippuric acid (PAH) 8, 15, 27, 44, 84, 92, 101
Passage time 69, 71
Penetration 71
–, rate of 72
Penicillin 92, 101
Pharmacogenetics 94
Phenobarbitone 95, 99
Phenol red 61

Phenylbutazone 47, 64, 65, 92
Phosphate 30
Pool 25
Potentiometer 106
Protein binding 6, 100
Pseudo-equilibrium 57

Quantities, fractional 50

Radio-immunoassay (RIA) 116
Rate, maintenance 33
Rate constant 107
– – of elimination 16
Reabsorption 8
–, gastrointestinal 7
–, tubular 94
Reaction, first-order 37
Regression, linear 14, 14
Regression coefficient 14
Renal failure 92
Residual functional capacity 91
Residuals 56

Salicyclates 92
Salicylamide 99
Saturation 17
Solvent deficiency 95
Sparteine 67
Steady-state 22, 58
–, analysis of 26

Steady-state concentration 24
Steroids 92
Streptomycin 92
Sulphonamides 48, 93, 95
Sulphonamidine 99
Suppository 47, 48, 48
Surface area 4
Systems, multicompartment 35, 67

Taylor series 125
Tetracyclines 15, 92, 128, 128
Tolbutamide 95
Total body water (TBW) 3
Transfer 29, 29
Transit 46
Treatment 62
Trial and error 110
Trick circuit 111, 112
Tubular secretion 9, 9

Vitamin A 81
Volume, total 58
– of distribution 1, 58, 102, 132
V_{ss} 59, 60

Water diuresis 95

Xanthinolnicotinate 99
Xylose 84

Kinetics of Drug Action

Editor: J. M. van Rossum

With contributions by J. Blanck, F. G. van den Brink, C. A. M. van Ginneken, R. E. Gosselin, P. T. Henderson, H. C. J. Ketelaars, E. Krüger-Thiemer, D. Mackay, J. M. van Rossum, W. Scheler, T. B. Vree

1977. 105 figures, 22 tables. XVII, 436 pages
(Handbook of Experimental Pharmacology, Vol. 47)
Cloth DM 220,– ; US $ 121.00
ISBN 3-540-08023-6

The contributions to this volume combine to make up an integrated presentation of the kinetics of drug action.

The fundamental aspects of transport processes across membranes relevant to drug transport are treated in the opening chapter. This is followed by a discussion of pharmacokinetics, including the kinetics of absorption, distribution, excretion and metabolism under linear and non-linear conditions. Drug schedules are discussed extensively. Drug-receptor interactions are treated in a further contribution. Another chapter presents a critical survey of current drug receptor theories.

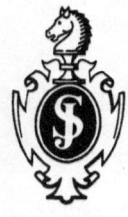

Contents: General Introduction. – Physiochemical Fundamentals and Thermodynamics of the Membrane Transport of Drugs. – Pharmacokinetics. Kinetic Aspects of Absorption, Distribution, and Elimination of Drugs. – Pharmacokinetics of Biotransformation. – General Theory of Drug-Receptor Interactions. Drug-Receptor Interaction Models. – Calculation of Drug Parameters. – A Critical Survey of Receptor Theories of Drug Action. – Drug-Receptor Inactivation: A New Kinetic Model. – Kinetics of Drug-Receptor Interaction. – Conclusion. – Author Index. – Subject Index.

Springer-Verlag
Berlin
Heidelberg
New York

Prices are subject to change without notice

Family Medicine: Principles and Practice

Editor: R. B. Taylor

Associate Editors: J. L. Buckingham, E. P. Donatelle W. E. Jacott, M. G. Rosen

1978. 204 figures. XXXIX, 1366 pages
Cloth DM 79,–; US $ 43.50
ISBN 3-540-90303-8

This is one of the most comprehensive textbooks of family medicine ever compiled. It is intended as a reference source of factual data about people in health and illness, presented as the approach of the family physician to clinical problems. There is a blend of fact and philosophy, theory and practice, and the book tells not only how to assess the familiy in crisis, calculate the fluid requirement of a person with serious burns, take a sexual history, and plan the diet for a diabetic, but also how to apply for hospital privileges, plan an office X-ray installation, and guide the patient to available community resources.

Discussed are the diagnosis and management of hundreds of clinical entities encompassing the full spectrum of health care, with guidelines to those problems the family physician should treat independently, share with a consultant, or refer for definitive care while providing a supportive role to the patient and family. Written for the family doctor, the book contains information useful for the medical student and vital for the practicing general practitioner.

Contents: The Family Physician. Family Medicine Education. Health Care Delivery. – The Patient. The Family. Behavior and Counseling. – Principles of Family Medicine: Clinical Evaluation. Clinical Approach to Problems. – Practice of Family Medicine: Planning for Family Practice. Facets of Family Practice. Interactions. Family Practice Today and Tomorrow.

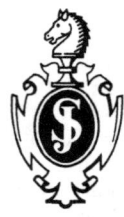

Springer-Verlag
Berlin
Heidelberg
New York

Prices are subject to change without notice

GPSR Compliance
The European Union's (EU) General Product Safety Regulation (GPSR) is a set of rules that requires consumer products to be safe and our obligations to ensure this.

If you have any concerns about our products, you can contact us on

ProductSafety@springernature.com

In case Publisher is established outside the EU, the EU authorized representative is:

Springer Nature Customer Service Center GmbH
Europaplatz 3
69115 Heidelberg, Germany

www.ingramcontent.com/pod-product-compliance
Lightning Source LLC
LaVergne TN
LVHW040740250326
834688LV00031B/379